Hypertension in Practice

Hypertension

in Practice

Third Edition

D Gareth Beevers MD FRCP
Professor of Medicine
City Hospital
Birmingham, UK

Graham A MacGregor FRCP
Professor of Cardiovascular Medicine
St George's Hospital Medical School
London, UK

MARTIN DUNITZ

Although every effort has been made to ensure that drug doses and other information are presented accurately in this publication, the ultimate responsibility rests with the prescribing physician. Neither the publishers nor the authors can be held responsible for errors or for any consequences arising from the use of information contained herein.

First published in the United Kingdom in 1987 by

Martin Dunitz Ltd
The Livery House
7–9 Pratt Street
London NW1 0AE

First edition 1987
First edition revised, paperback 1988
Second edition 1995
Third edition 1999

A CIP catalogue record for this book is available from the British Library

ISBN 1–85317–591–9

Distributed in the United States by:
Blackwell Science Inc.
Commerce Place, 350 Main Street
Malden, MA 02148, USA
Tel: 1-800-215-1000

Composition by Scribe Design, Gillingham, Kent
Printed and bound in Spain

CONTENTS

ACKNOWLEDGEMENTS

We are immensely grateful to Dr Emma Baker from St George's Hospital, London for detailed criticisms and advice and Dr Frances Aitchison from the Department of Radiology, City Hospital, Birmingham for advice on radiological investigations.

PREFACE TO THE THIRD EDITION

This third edition, so soon after the second, became necessary because of advances in medical knowledge. The publication in 1997 of the SYST-EUR trial was an important event. It was the first mortality and morbidity trial to examine the value of the "newer" classes of antihypertensive drugs, and the benefits of treatment were impressive. This study was also able to reassure us that the anxieties about the possible long-term hazards of calcium-channel blockers may have been groundless.

In 1998, the Hypertension Optimal Treatment (HOT) trial was published. This large study investigated the so-called J curve and gave us reliable information on how far we should lower blood pressure with drugs. This trial also investigated the value of aspirin.

The other main event prompting us to produce the third edition was the impressive success of the angiotensin-receptor antagonists, a new and very interesting class of antihypertensive drugs with remarkably few side-effects and possibly some added benefits.

Sadly, however, the Health Survey for England has shown us that there is still a depressing state of underdiagnosis and undertreatment of hypertension in the community. Anything we can do to increase awareness of this shortfall of delivery of validated treatment for hypertension is worthwhile.

Perhaps the success of this book so far has been related to our decision to provide a readable and clear account of the management of hypertension. We have not attempted to produce a textbook including every fine detail of the various syndromes of hypertension as there are many excellent volumes where details can be found and references obtained. This book is designed to be read rather than referred to and the reader has to accept that this is our interpretation of the word literature and of current opinions together with our largely documented experience based on the management of thousands of patients.

D Gareth Beevers
Graham A MacGregor

1

Section One

1 THE IMPORTANCE OF HYPERTENSION

BACKGROUND

High blood pressure or hypertension is now the most common chronic medical condition in the developed world. Depending on the criteria for the diagnosis, it can be said to be present in 20–30% of the adult population. Furthermore, it is rapidly becoming a major problem in the developing countries.

Hypertension should not be regarded so much as a disease (although some patients may be clinically unwell) but more as one of three treatable or reversible risk factors for premature death due to arterial disease. In this chapter, the structural lesions in the blood vessels that are either a cause of, or are caused by, hypertension are described. We also examine the effects of these vascular lesions on the heart and brain in what may be termed 'end-organ' or 'target-organ' damage.

In general, the amount of end-organ damage is directly proportional to the height of the blood pressure, and this gradient of risk extends down into the range of blood pressure that is conventionally described as 'normal'. Thus, an individual with a diastolic blood pressure of 80 mmHg is at greater risk of cardiovascular disease than a similar individual with a diastolic blood pressure of 70 mmHg, although neither of these individuals would be considered to be hypertensive. The first individual has a measurably higher blood pressure and this difference in pressure is explicable on the basis of a higher peripheral vascular resistance.

THE BLOOD VESSELS IN HYPERTENSION

Peripheral resistance

The elevation of blood pressure in hypertensive patients is directly related to the degree of peripheral arteriolar narrowing (peripheral vascular resistance). In essential hypertension, the cardiac output is normal until end-organ cardiac damage causes it to fall. This peripheral arteriolar narrowing is due to two closely interlocking factors.

1. Arteriolar smooth muscle constriction
2. Growth and proliferation of arteriolar smooth muscle cells.

The factors causing this vasoconstriction and vascular growth are described in more detail in Chapter 4. The other lesions of small and large blood vessels are described in detail here (Fig. 1.1).

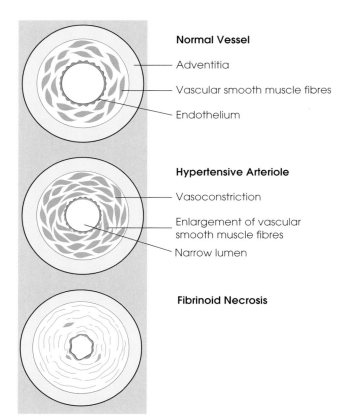

Normal Vessel

Adventitia

Vascular smooth muscle fibres

Endothelium

Hypertensive Arteriole

Vasoconstriction

Enlargement of vascular smooth muscle fibres

Narrow lumen

Fibrinoid Necrosis

Figure 1.1
The arteriolar lesions of hypertension.

Arteriolar fibroid hyaline necrosis

Arteriolar fibroid hyaline necrosis is the hallmark of accelerated or malignant phase hypertension. Microvascular necroses are found in the arterioles of the brain, heart, kidneys, retina and many other sites but not in skeletal muscle or skin.

Arteriolar thickening

As described earlier, arteriolar thickening is the basic lesion of hypertension leading to the increased peripheral vascular resistance.

There is realignment of smooth muscle cells, which are also larger than normal, and in vivo are relatively constricted. As the external diameter of these arterioles is also slightly reduced, the internal (luminal) diameter is greatly reduced so peripheral resistance is increased.

Atheroma

Hypertensive patients are particularly prone to develop atheroma in larger blood vessels due to lipid-rich deposits in the arterial wall. Cigarette smoking and hyperlipidaemia also

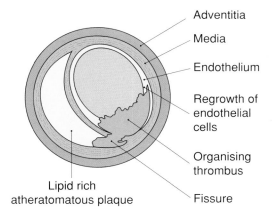

Adventitia

Media

Endothelium

Regrowth of endothelial cells

Organising thrombus

Fissure

Lipid rich atheratomatous plaque

Figure 1.2
Schematic cross-section of an artery showing fissuring of an atheromatous plaque with intravascular thrombosis.

increase this rate of deposition. Atheroma is particularly prominent in regions of haemodynamic turbulence where blood vessels divide. Also, high blood pressure facilitates fissuring of the atheromatous plaque, which leads to further atheroma, related to platelet adhesion and cholesterol incorporation (Fig. 1.2). Atheroma causes patchy or confluent narrowing of cerebral and coronary arteries as well as of the aorta and leg arteries. In the renal arteries, this can cause atheromatous renal artery stenosis. Hypertensive patients with very low plasma cholesterol levels are much less prone to develop atheroma although they still do develop the haemorrhagic complications of raised blood pressure.

Intravascular thrombosis

There is a tendency for intravascular thrombosis to develop in atheromatous vessels,

particularly in the cerebral and coronary circulations. This may lead to complete occlusion of the vessel with infarction of the tissues supplied by that vessel. There is evidence that people with raised blood pressure have a greater tendency to intravascular thrombosis partly because of increased platelet activation, raised plasma fibrinogen levels and an increased platelet–vessel wall interaction.

Aneurysm

Large vessel saccular or fusiform aneurysms are commoner in hypertensive patients, who thus have an increased chance of developing both aortic dissection, either in the abdomen or the thorax, and abdominal aneurysms containing thrombus.

Charcot–Bouchard aneurysms

Microvascular aneurysms of the intracerebral arteries, named after Charcot and Bouchard, are almost specific to hypertension. When they rupture, they cause intracerebral haemorrhage.

Berry aneurysms

Aneurysms of the circle of Willis are common in severe hypertension, particularly if this is due to autosomal dominant polycystic kidney disease. Their rupture leads to sub-arachnoid haemorrhage.

Fibromuscular hyperplasia

Renal artery narrowing in younger hypertensive patients may be due to fibromuscular hyperplasia. The arteries assume an irregular 'string of beads' appearance. In children, this may also be seen in the mesenteric and other abdominal arteries. When the renal arteries are affected, this is a cause rather than the consequence of the hypertension; the aetiology is unknown but it is commoner in women. This condition should not be confused with atheromatous renal artery stenosis, a condition seen in older patients, particularly if they are smokers.

VASCULAR END-ORGAN DAMAGE

The heart

Left ventricular hypertrophy

Clinical, radiological, ECG or echocardiographic evidence of left ventricular hypertrophy (LVH) is closely correlated to the height of the blood pressure (Fig. 1.3). About 50% of patients with moderate hypertension (diastolic pressures of 110–120 mmHg) have the ECG criteria for definite LVH. There is some evidence that LVH is not solely due to the degree of elevation of blood pressure but may be related to circulating growth factors, particularly angiotensin, and a direct effect of these hormones that also elevate blood pressure. When LVH is present, the prognosis is bad. A hypertensive patient with LVH has four times the chance of developing a heart attack compared with a patient with a similar level of blood pressure but no LVH. Such patients also have an increased risk of thrombotic stroke (suggesting a prothrombotic tendency) and a three-fold higher risk of intermittent claudication. For this reason, a routine ECG in a new hypertensive patient is a very powerful predictor of outcome. Whilst the ECG features of LVH are reason-

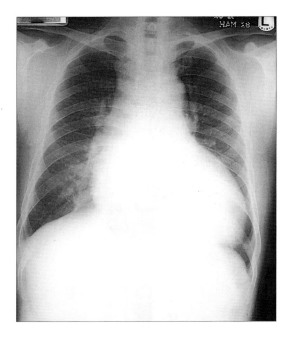

Figure 1.3
Chest X–ray showing cardiomegaly due to severe hypertension.

ably specific, they are not very sensitive. Thus, hypertrophy may be present even if the ECG is normal. Echocardiography is a more sensitive method of detecting LVH but this test is not generally available in routine practice.

Hypertensive patients with large left ventricles are more prone to cardiac arrhythmias, particularly if they have hypokalaemia related to high-dose diuretic therapy.

Myocardial infarction

Coronary heart disease is twice as common in hypertensive patients than in the remainder of the population (Fig. 1.4). The risk of

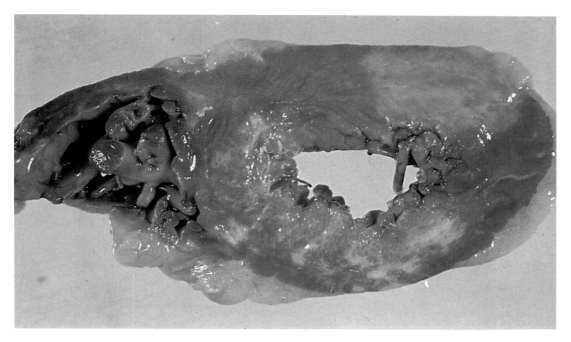

Figure 1.4
Hypertrophied left ventricle with pale wedge–shaped myocardial infarction in a patient with severe hypertension.

heart attack is directly related to the height of the blood pressure. About 1% of all hypertensive patients suffer a myocardial infarction each year, whereas the figure is only about half this for people with diastolic blood pressures below 90 mmHg. The incidence of myocardial infarction in patients with uncontrolled hypertension rises to 3% per year, and this increases further if other risk factors are present. A patient with myocardial infarction and pre-existing hypertension has a worse prognosis than a similar patient with no such history. Hypertensive patients who also smoke cigarettes have an even worse prognosis, particularly from sudden death, their risk being about twice as much again. Similarly, the risk is increased if there are also raised plasma cholesterol levels particularly with low HDL cholesterol levels (see Chapter 2).

Angina pectoris

Angina is about twice as common in hypertensive patients than in normotensives. This may partly be due to atheroma of coronary arteries, causing ischaemia, but it may also be compounded by the relatively larger left ventricular mass with no corresponding increase in the blood supply. Lowering the blood pressure may relieve angina even if drugs without antianginal activity are used. Exercise tests according to the Bruce protocol

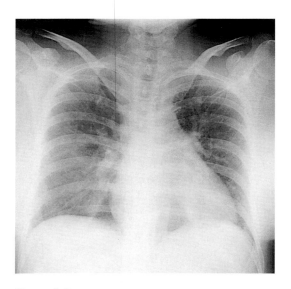

Figure 1.5
Chest X–ray showing cardiomegaly with
pulmonary oedema and marked upper lobe
diversion.

and 24-hour ECGs demonstrate an increased
frequency of symptomless ECG changes of
ischaemia in hypertensive patients, even
though coronary angiography may demonstrate remarkably little atheroma.

Heart failure

Heart failure is four times more common in
hypertensive women and seven times more
common in hypertensive men in comparison
with age- and sex-matched normotensive
people, and the risk rises with advancing age.
Left ventricular failure may occur in a hypertensive patient following a myocardial infarction but may also develop in hypertensives
who have LVH alone (Fig. 1.5). This form of
heart failure should, therefore, be preventable

if blood pressures are well controlled. In the
ageing population, frequently with poorly
controlled hypertension, heart failure is
becoming more common. More patients with
acute myocardial infarction now survive the
immediate event but tend to develop heart
failure in later life.

Cardiomyopathy

Some hypertensive patients with big, poorly
contracting hearts and dilatation of all four
cardiac chambers, often with atrial fibrillation, may be heavy alcohol consumers. High
alcohol intake can cause a congestive
cardiomyopathy as well as hypertension.
There is no convincing evidence of the
existence of a syndrome of 'hypertensive
cardiomyopathy'.

The brain

Subarachnoid haemorrhage

About 50% of patients with subarachnoid
haemorrhage have pre-existing hypertension,
and about 30% do not have berry aneurysms
of the circle of Willis. Cigarette smoking is
also closely associated with subarachnoid
haemorrhage. When a vessel ruptures, the
patient develops acute meningeal irritation
with severe headache and usually rapid loss
of consciousness. About half of all patients die
after their first haemorrhage, but this figure
may be reduced by surgical clipping of an
aneurysm and with the control of hypertension. There is evidence that the calcium-
channel blocker, nimodipine, reduces the risk
of a second subarachnoid haemorrhage and,
similarly, some evidence of benefit from
beta-adrenergic blockade. However, rapid
reductions of blood pressure may be

L R

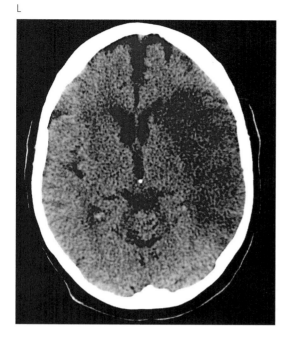

Figure 1.6
CT scan showing large cerebral infarct in the right cerebral cortex.

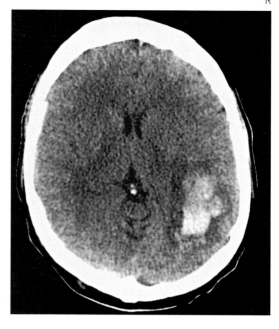

Figure 1.7
CT scan showing right intracerebral haemorrhage.

hazardous to those areas of the brain close to the ruptured blood vessel. Intracerebral arteries may exhibit intense spasm, leading to a reduction in cerebral blood flow. Nimodipine may reduce this spasm but over-rapid reduction of blood pressure could make this situation worse.

Cerebral infarcts

In hypertensive patients, the most common cerebral lesion is a cerebral infarction (Fig. 1.6). This is related to cerebral thrombosis associated with atheroma of the intracranial vessels. The overall risk of the development of a stroke in a hypertensive man is about one-quarter of the risk of developing a myocardial infarction. The incidence is about 2% per year in patients with diastolic blood pressures around 110 mmHg. In mild hypertension, where diastolic pressures are around 100 mmHg, the incidence is 0.5% per year. Of patients under the age of 70 years admitted to hospital with stroke, about half have pre-existing hypertension. There is evidence to suggest that high alcohol intake and cigarette smoking are important precipitating factors causing premature stroke. This may be due to an acute rise in blood

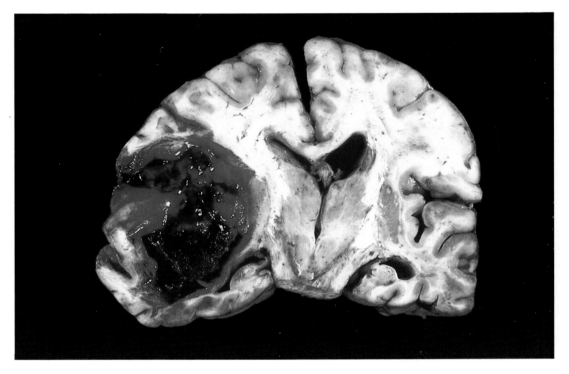

Figure 1.8
Brain showing intracerebral haemorrhage.

pressure following heavy drinking or possibly to alcohol- or nicotine-induced cerebral vasoconstriction. Serum cholesterol levels are also a weak risk factor for strokes as is the presence of concomitant diabetes mellitus. More recently, studies have strongly suggested that a high salt intake may predispose to stroke, independently of blood pressure, suggesting a direct effect of salt in vessel walls.

Cerebral haemorrhage

The more frequent use of CT scanning in patients who have sustained a stroke has

demonstrated that cerebral haemorrhage is not, in fact, the commonest cerebral complication of hypertension (Figs 1.7 and 1.8). Previously, if a hypertensive patient developed a stroke it was assumed that this was due to a cerebral haemorrhage as a result of high pressure in the intracerebral microaneurysms of Charcot and Bouchard. Again, cigarette smoking is an important added risk factor.

Cerebral embolus

Embolisation can occur from a left ventricular thrombus in patients following a myocardial infarction or from a left atrial thrombus in patients with atrial fibrillation with or without mitral stenosis. Another source of embolus is from atheromatous carotid artery stenosis. The clinical presentation is either of a transient cerebral ischaemic attack (TIA) or of a completed stroke. Both are commoner in patients with high blood pressure, particularly if there is associated LVH.

Cerebral blood flow

In normal circumstances, the blood flow to the brain is remarkably constant despite fluctuations in blood pressure. This state of cerebral 'autoregulation', however, breaks down with very high or very low blood pressure or following a stroke. When blood pressure is reduced rapidly by more than about 35%, cerebral blood flow falls and further cerebral ischaemia may develop. When blood pressures are very high (for example, a diastolic blood pressure of 140 mmHg or more), cerebral blood flow rises and cerebral oedema may develop, leading to the clinical state of hypertensive encephalopathy. In hypertensive patients, cerebral autoregulation is reset at a slightly higher level and blood flow remains constant as long as pressures are not lowered too rapidly.

Encephalopathy

The syndrome of hypertensive encephalopathy is very rare but it may be seen in association with the malignant or accelerated phase of hypertension. If a hypertensive patient develops a sudden onset of focal neurological deficit, it is most likely to be due to a stroke and, under these circumstances, rapid reduction of blood pressure can be dangerous. Very rarely, focal neuro-

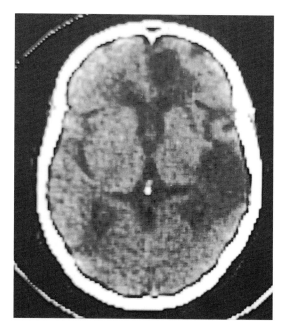

Figure 1.9
CT scan showing multiple cerebral infarcts in a patient with dementia.

logical signs may develop in a very severely hypertensive patient where there is no cerebral infarct or haemorrhage. The syndrome of encephalopathy is almost impossible to diagnose without performing a CT scan to exclude a structural cerebral lesion. Encephalopathy may be considered if there are fluctuating neurological signs with restlessness, confusion and sometimes generalised convulsions. Here, rapid but controlled reduction of blood pressure is necessary, often with intravenous drugs.

Lacunae

There is now increasing evidence from CT scanning that many hypertensive patients

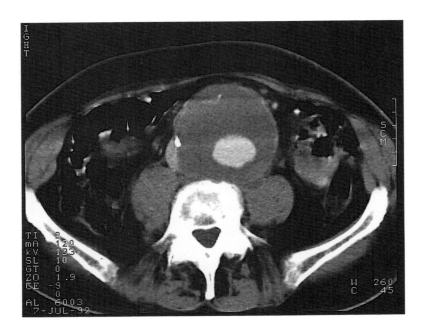

Figure 1.10
CT scan showing large abdominal aortic aneurysm with extensive intravascular thrombosis and narrow lumen containing contrast medium.

with no focal neurological signs do have small intracerebral neurological lesions (Fig. 1.9). Clinically, these patients may have memory impairment with reduction of cognitive skills. More extreme cases are encountered when hypertension is associated with general deterioration of cerebral function, dementia, hyper-reflexia and a steadily downward clinical progress. This syndrome of multi-infarct dementia is sometimes referred to as 'Binswanger's disease'.

The peripheral vessels

Aneurysm

Atheromatous plaques develop in the aorta and may progress to aortic aneurysm or aortic dissection (Fig. 1.10). Death from rupture of an aortic aneurysm is three times commoner in hypertensive patients than in normotensives.

Intermittent claudication

Intermittent claudication is twice as frequent in hypertensive patients than in people with normal blood pressure. The other cardio-vascular risk factors, cigarette smoking and hyperlipidaemia, are often present. It should be remembered that beta-blockers, used to control blood pressure, may induce or aggravate claudication in patients with pre-existing peripheral vascular disease.

Many patients with peripheral vascular disease may also have previously undiag-nosed atheromatous renal artery stenosis, which may be contributing to the hyperten-

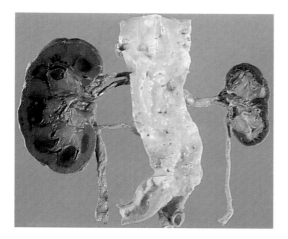

Figure 1.11
Aortic atheroma and left renal artery stenosis.
(Reproduced with permission from Swales JD,
Sever PS, Peart S. *Clinical Atlas of Hypertension.*
Gower Medical Publishing, 1991; Fig. 5.10.)

sion and renal impairment (Fig. 1.11). Atheromatous renal artery stenosis is also seen in normotensive patients with peripheral vascular disease, particularly if they are smokers.

The kidney

Hypertensive nephrosclerosis

Mild symptomless haematuria and proteinuria are common in hypertension even when this is not associated with the malignant/accelerated phase or evidence of an underlying intrinsic renal disease. When proteinuria is present, shown by dipstick testing, the mortality rate from vascular complications for hypertension is approximately doubled. Similarly, in hypertensive patients with a serum urea level of 10 mmol/l, the mortality is twice that of patients with no renal impairment. Uncontrolled severe hypertension causes progressive renal damage, and irreversible renal failure may develop. The overall risk of developing chronic renal failure in hypertensive patients is about five times higher than in normotensive patients with renal damage. There remains, however, some debate as to whether non-malignant essential mild hypertension can cause kidney failure. Whilst there is no doubt that mild hypertension does cause heart attacks and strokes, there does not appear to be an increased risk of developing renal failure. If a mildly hypertensive patient has proteinuria or evidence of renal impairment, then often some underlying renal disease may be present that may have initiated the raised blood pressure, and a vicious cycle may follow where hypertension causes further renal damage.

Hypertension is present in 70% of patients undergoing chronic renal dialysis. Furthermore, hypertension complicates up to 70% of cases with intrinsic renal disease, including various forms of glomerulonephritis.

Renal artery stenosis

Atheromatous renal artery narrowing or occlusion may occur as a consequence of high blood pressure in older patients, particularly if they are smokers. It is, however, worth diagnosing and treating, as surgical repair of the renal artery or angioplasty may reduce the blood pressure or make it easier to control with drugs and may also lead to some preservation of renal function.

In younger patients, renal artery stenosis may be due to fibromuscular hyperplasia of the renal arteries, and surgery or angioplasty may lead to normalisation of the blood pressure.

Atheromatous or fibrodysplastic renal artery stenosis goes undiagnosed unless angiography or isotope renography is undertaken. Older hypertensive patients with evidence of arterial disease elsewhere (claudication, femoral or carotid bruits) may have renal artery stenosis, which may influence the choice of antihypertensive drugs.

MALIGNANT HYPERTENSION

Malignant and accelerated hypertension are now considered to be the same condition as their aetiology, prognosis and treatment are the same. Malignant hypertension is a multisystem disorder, characterised by arteriolar fibrinoid necrosis. Death is usually due to progressive renal failure, heart failure or stroke. If left untreated, most patients die within 2 years. Whilst renal or adrenal causes of hypertension frequently underlie the malignant phase, about 65% of cases still have essential rather than secondary hypertension. Malignant hypertension is closely associated with cigarette smoking.

The ophthalmological features of malignant hypertension are retinal flame-shaped haemorrhages, cotton wool spots and hard exudates, particularly forming a macular star, and there may or may not be papilloedema. Patients who have all retinal features except papilloedema were once labelled accelerated hypertensives but this distinction is now obsolete.

As part of this multisystem disorder, microangiopathic haemolytic anaemia may be seen, whereas this is not seen in non-malignant hypertension unless there is severe renal failure. Some patients with malignant hypertension do not have cardiomegaly, even on echocardiography, implying that not all cases are due to longstanding hypertension but may instead have a relatively acute onset. The incidence of malignant phase hypertension appears to be declining, possibly as a result of the more efficient detection and management of hypertension in its earlier stages. Many patients present with visual symptoms, which results in their first presenting to an ophthalmologist.

MULTIPLE RISK FACTORS

As stated earlier, hypertension must be seen as one of three cardiovascular risk factors, and in clinical practice all these factors need attention. Chapter 2 enlarges upon the concept of multiple risk and discusses recent advances in our understanding of the epidemiology of hypertension.

FURTHER READING

Bamford J, Sandercock P, Dennis M, et al. Classification of natural history of clinically identifiable subtypes of cerebral infarction. Lancet 1991; **337**: 1521–6.

Davies MJ, Woolf N, Rowles PM, et al. Morphology of the endothelium over atherosclerotic plaques in human coronary arteries. Br Heart J 1988; **60**: 459–64.

Folkow B, Grimsby G, Thulesius OE. Adaptive structural changes of the vascular walls in hypertension and their relation to the control of the peripheral resistance. Acta Physiol Scand 1958; **44**: 252–72.

Lip GYH, Gammage MD, Beevers DG. Hypertension in the heart. Br Med Bull 1994; **50**: 299–321.

Pulsinelli W. Pathophysiology of acute ischaemic stroke. Lancet 1992; **339**: 533–6.

Raine AEG. Hypertension and the kidney. Br Med Bull 1994; **50**: 322–41.

2 HYPERTENSION AND CARDIOVASCULAR RISK

BACKGROUND

In terms of life expectancy, as well as mortality and morbidity, the height of the blood pressure must be seen in the context of other important reversible cardio-vascular risk factors such as raised plasma lipid levels and cigarette smoking. In this chapter, the multiple risk factor approach to hypertension is enlarged upon. Also discussed is the magnitude of this risk to the individual and to populations. The chapter opens with a series of definitions of hypertension which, though arbitrary, are relevant to clinical medicine and to epidemiology. Finally, we draw attention to the fact that a great many hypertensive patients, who have levels of blood pressure that definitely require treatment, remain undiagnosed, and even if diagnosed many are untreated or undertreated.

THE DEFINITION OF HYPERTENSION

In the last 30 years, the importance of hypertension as a cause of heart attacks and strokes has become increasingly recognised, largely because of the advent of acceptable antihypertensive drugs. However, the continuing confusion as to the criteria for diagnosing hypertension may be attributed to the fact that there is still no universally recognised definition of the condition. Attempts to provide a universal definition have so far been unsuccessful. Given below is a pragmatic view relevant to clinical practice, although the epidemiological view also requires detailed consideration.

The pragmatic definition of hypertension

The late Professor Geoffrey Rose suggested that the best clinical definition of hypertension should be 'that level of blood pressure above which investigation and treatment do more good than harm'. When following this pragmatic approach the clinician must be fully up to date with the published clinical trials on the usefulness of the treatment of hypertension in a field where new information is constantly becoming available. This definition may change as more trials are completed. Over the last 10 years the pragmatic definition of hypertension, particularly in the elderly, has changed substantially following the publication of a series of well-conducted randomised controlled trials.

The current pragmatic definition of diastolic hypertension is a diastolic blood pressure, in patients below the age of 80 years, measured at the fifth phase (disappearance of diastolic sounds), which after four clinical examinations exceeds 90 mmHg. Over the age of 80 years, there is less clarity as to the level where treatment is worthwhile, but hypertension might then be defined as a diastolic blood pressure persistently greater than 100 mmHg when measured under the same conditions. Patients whose blood pressures are at or above these levels need elementary investigation and follow-up and, in more severe cases, detailed tests to identify underlying causes. Below these blood pressure levels, drug therapy has not been shown to be useful. In some cases it might even be harmful because of the anxiety or distress caused to patients and the side-effects of antihypertensive drugs, with only minimal benefits in terms of coronary or stroke prevention. The WHO criteria (Table 2.1) have the disadvantage that they do not take into account the individual's age, or the number of times the pressure is measured.

Isolated systolic hypertension

The foregoing definition takes no account of the height of the systolic blood pressure. Recent impressive evidence shows that elevated systolic blood pressures are worth treating even when the diastolic blood pressures are unequivocally normal. Epidemiologists have long considered that the concentration on the part of clinicians on the diastolic blood pressure alone is not logical. Population surveys and studies of hypertensive patients have shown that the height of systolic blood pressure is usually

Table 2.1
Definitions of hypertension (WHO criteria)

Normal	Systolic BP less than 140 mmHg and diastolic BP less than 90 mmHg
Borderline	Systolic BP 140–159 mmHg and/or diastolic BP 90–94 mmHg
Hypertension	Systolic BP 160 mmHg or more and/or diastolic BP 95 mmHg or more
Mild Hypertension	Systolic BP 160–179 mmHg and/or diastolic BP 95–104 mmHg
Isolated Systolic Hypertension (ISH)	Systolic BP 160 mmHg or more and diastolic BP below 95 mmHg

a better predictor of death than the height of the diastolic blood pressure. For example, it is possible to calculate from insurance company data that a man aged 35 with a blood pressure of 160/90 has a shorter life expectancy than a similar man whose blood pressure is 150/100, if left untreated. Although the diastolic blood pressure of the former is lower, his higher systolic blood pressure means that he is at greater risk.

The main reason why elevation of systolic blood pressure has a greater prognostic value that of the diastolic blood pressure is because systolic pressure rises more sharply with advancing age, and this rise may, in part, be caused by the development of thickening of the large arteries due to chronically raised intra-arterial pressure. This implies that raised systolic blood pressure may, in some respects, be a reflection of arterial damage. The presence of other evidence of end-organ damage, for example left ventricular hypertrophy (LVH) or a previous vascular complication, such as a stroke, is, not surprisingly, a powerful prognostic feature in an individual patient. It might be inferred, therefore, that the level of systolic blood pressure would be more closely related to life expectancy than the diastolic blood pressure.

In the elderly, the systolic blood pressure, which is mainly related to a continuing rise in peripheral resistance, rises steadily with advancing age and continues to predict life expectancy accurately. By contrast, after about the age of 60 years, diastolic blood pressures tend to level off and then fall gradually, possibly due to a decline in cardiac output. This explains, at least in part, why the height of the diastolic blood pressure is less predictive over the age of about 60 years.

BLOOD PRESSURE IN POPULATIONS

An understanding of the epidemiological approach to blood pressure is important to the clinician if he or she is to manage hyper-

tensive patients properly. The epidemiologist sees blood pressure from the point of view of its impact on the health of the whole population rather than of individual patients. Sir George Pickering pointed out that hypertension should be seen as a quantitative rather than a qualitative entity. In the general population, blood pressure is distributed in a roughly normal or Gaussian manner in a bell-shaped curve with a slight skew towards higher readings (Fig. 2.1). There is, therefore, no evidence for any subgroup of hypertensive individuals distinct from normotensives, and no dividing line can be identified between normal and raised blood pressure levels.

Pickering also drew attention to the fact that the risk of heart attack or stroke is directly related to the height of blood pressure at all levels. Even people whose blood pressures are average or even below average for their age have a higher cardiovascular risk than those with lower pressures, although they would not be regarded as clinically hypertensive (Fig. 2.2). Hypertension appears to be a disease of

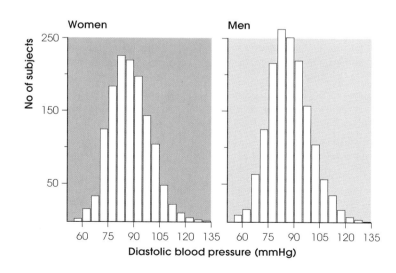

Figure 2.1

The distribution of blood pressure in middle-aged men and women attending nine general practitioners in Renfrew, Scotland.

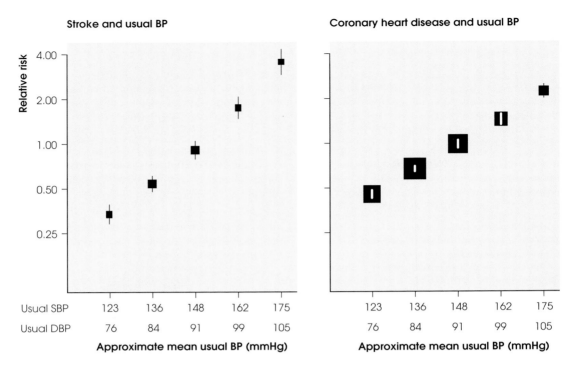

Figure 2.2
The relative risks of stroke and heart attack in relation to systolic and diastolic blood pressures. Pooled data from nine study populations. The size of the boxes gives an indication of the number of cardiovascular events.

quantity rather than of quality and the higher the pressure the worse the outlook. There is no dividing line between pressures that carry a low risk and pressures that are associated with premature death.

It is apparent that, with the exception of hypotension due to autonomic neuropathy or severe generalised illness, Addison's disease or following a heart attack, it is not possible to have blood pressure that is too low. Unlike hypertension, which is associated with premature death, low blood pressure on its own is not a diagnosis of any prognostic significance, even though there are reports that individuals with low pressures may have a higher frequency of depression and non-specific mild complaints. This association is probably due to a tendency of such patients to lose weight due to anorexia, but, despite these symptoms, they tend to live longer.

BLOOD PRESSURE AND AGE

In Westernised societies, average blood pressures tend to rise with advancing age. This rise starts soon after birth and

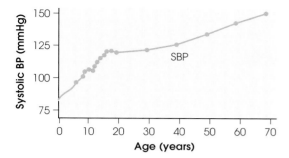

Figure 2.3
Changes in systolic blood pressure with age.

continues until the age of about 6 weeks. Blood pressures then level off until about the age of 4 years. They then start to rise again and continue to do so up until the age of about 60 with a particularly sharp rise during the growth spurt of adolescence (Fig. 2.3). This phenomenon is not seen in most primitive or rural populations where, consequently, hypertension and its vascular complications are very rare. Thus, the epidemiologist would prefer to see action taken to prevent this rise in the first place, as this could lead to effective primary prevention of hypertension, and its cardiovascular complications. The rise in blood pressure with age is not 'normal' or physiological and its avoidance would be beneficial to the health of the nation.

THE PUBLIC HEALTH APPROACH

The public health physician considers that 'clinical' hypertension is a disease affecting varying numbers of people who are, epidemiologically speaking, not particularly important or common. Instead, the epidemiologist considers that blood pressures of the whole population in Westernised societies are too high and that these pressures explain the high incidence of heart attack and stroke. If the average blood pressure of the population could be reduced by as little as 5 mmHg, then there should be a reduction of the heart attack and stroke rates in the whole population by an amount greater than could be achieved by the efficient detection and management of all 'clinically' hypertensive patients.

The concept of personal risk versus population risk may, at first, sound mutually exclusive but this is not so. Within the concept of improving primary health care, as well as managing those individuals with 'clinical' hypertension, the 'high-risk' strategy and the 'whole population' approach can be carried out simultaneously. General practitioners (GPs) should therefore have a responsibility for the blood pressure of all of their patients, not just those with levels above the threshold for starting antihypertensive therapy.

COMPLICATIONS OF HYPERTENSION

High blood pressure has been called the silent killer as it is usually symptomless until an advanced stage. One disastrous definition of hypertension is based solely on the symptoms or complications of the disease, which means that treatment is not started until there is evidence of target organ damage. If this definition alone were to be employed, then the population would suffer even more potentially preventable strokes, heart attacks and other vascular crises than it does at present. Only about 30% of hypertensive patients have evidence of cardiovascular disease when first detected in a primary health care setting. It is far too late to wait for ECG evidence of LVH, yet alone clinical evidence of angina, heart attack or stroke.

Malignant hypertension

The term malignant hypertension is now regarded as being synonymous with accelerated hypertension. It implies very high blood pressures in association with retinal haemorrhages, exudates, and cotton wool spots with or without papilloedema. If left untreated, 88% of such cases die within 2 years. Malignant hypertension can be either 'essential' or secondary to some underlying disease.

Benign hypertension

Benign hypertension is an unfortunate term that is best avoided. It simply means that the hypertension is not associated with malignant hypertensive retinopathy. However, the prognosis of 'benign' hypertension in its severer forms can hardly be regarded as benign.

Primary or essential hypertension

The term primary hypertension is reserved for the 95% of hypertensive patients, in whom no immediately evident underlying renal or adrenal cause can be found for the raised blood pressure. It is a confusing term

as clearly all hypertension does have a cause, even if this is due to complicated inter-relationships between genetic and environmental factors.

Secondary hypertension

In a minority of hypertensive patients, the raised blood pressure is due to underlying renal or renal artery disease, adrenal cortical or medullary hormone excess, drugs or systemic arteritis (see Chapters 4 and 8).

How common is hypertension

In men and women aged 35–65 years of age, severe hypertension with diastolic pressures of 130 mmHg or more is found in about 0.5% of the population (Table 2.2). A small proportion of these patients may have the malignant phase of hypertension. This syndrome is, however, fortunately rare. In a

Table 2.2
Estimated number of patients who are registered with an average UK general practice who have a single casual blood pressure of 160/95 mm Hg or more. Figures in brackets denote the percentage of people in that age band with hypertension.

Age	Men	Women
0–19	7 (2%)	4 (1%)
20–39	25 (7%)	8 (3%)
40–59	70 (25%)	52 (18%)
60–79	66 (35%)	93 (37%)
80+	10 (50%)	26 (50%)
Total	178	183

busy district hospital serving a population of around 300,000 people, about five or six new cases of malignant hypertension are seen each year.

Diastolic blood pressures of 110–129 mmHg are found in about 4% of the adult Caucasian population and 8–9% of blacks in the UK and the USA. These figures show that in whites this disease has about twice the prevalence of diabetes mellitus.

The combined prevalence of moderate and severe hypertension is, therefore, around 4.5%. In the average primary health care practice, with about 2000 patients of all ages registered with a single GP, about 15 patients below the age of 65 will be found to have diastolic blood pressures of 110 mmHg or more.

It can be seen from the bell-shaped curve of the distribution of blood pressure (Fig 2.1) that the milder grades of hypertension are the most common. Diastolic blood pressures between 90 and 109 mmHg are found in about 20% of the middle-aged adult population. In younger adults the prevalence is lower, and in the elderly the prevalence is correspondingly higher. A casual blood pressure of 160/95 mmHg or more is found in roughly 50% of Western populations aged 70 years or more (Fig. 2.4). It is possible to calculate that in the population of England and Wales (roughly 50 million people), 7,196,000 people (14.5% of the population) of all ages will have a single casual blood pressure reading of this level or above. An average GP should, therefore, expect to have around 300 patients on his list with a single casual blood pressure reading of 160/95 mmHg or more.

Similarly, in the USA, blood pressures exceeding 160/95 mmHg have been estimated to be present in 23.2 million people, this representing 15–19% of whites and 27–29% of blacks aged 18–74. If the criteria for diagnosing hypertension are

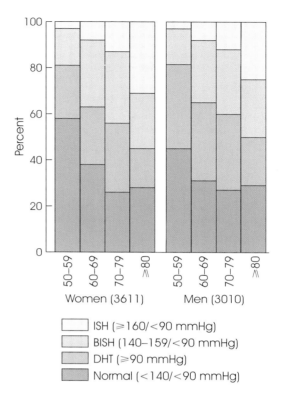

Figure 2.4

Prevalence of systolic and diastolic hypertension in the Copenhagen City Heart Study. (*J Hum Hypertens* 1995; **9**: 175–80.)
ISH, Isolated systolic hypertension
BISH, Borderline isolated systolic hypertension
DHT, Diastolic hypertension

lowered to include cases with diastolic pressures between 90 and 95 mmHg, then around 40% of the population may be considered hypertensive. Isolated systolic hypertension (ISH), where systolic pressures exceed 160 mmHg whilst diastolic pressures are below 95 mmHg, is found in around 5% of people aged under 60 years, but in around 25% of people aged 75 years. This latter group are known to benefit from antihypertensive therapy. The above figures, obtained from population screening surveys, are based on single casual blood pressure readings. On rechecking, many of these high blood pressures will settle. This is partly due to familiarisation of individuals to the screening techniques, and partly due to the statistical trend for initially high values (and initially low values) to move towards the mean of the population on resampling. After measuring blood pressure on three or four occasions, the prevalence of hypertension falls. In one recent American study, only 6.9% of the non-elderly population had diastolic blood pressures that were persistently 90 mmHg or over.

All the above statistics were based on population surveys that have employed diastolic blood pressures measured at the disappearance of sounds (fifth phase). A higher prevalence would be found if the muffling of sound (fourth phase) were used, although this technique is now considered obsolete. Variations between different population surveys may be due to differences in diastolic endpoints, and also to the number of readings taken, and the age, gender and ethnic distribution of the population under study. Other factors influencing pressures are the manometer cuff size and the position of the arm in relation to the heart, the amount of training of the observers, the time of day and time of year, the ambient temperature, the anxiety of the subject, and the wait time before the pressure is actually measured (see Chapter 3).

THE RISK OF HYPERTENSION

High blood pressure is the commonest risk factor for the most prevalent cause of death in Western populations. The 2-year survival rate for patients with malignant

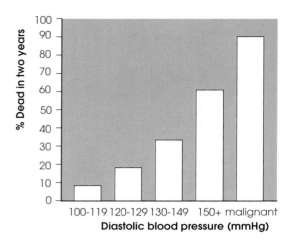

Figure 2.5

Mortality rate for untreated patients with high blood pressure. Data from AWD Leishman, Sheffield, 1959.

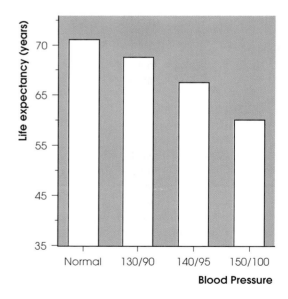

Figure 2.6

Life expectancy in relation to untreated blood pressure in men aged 35 years. Data from the Metropolitan Life Insurance Company, 1961.

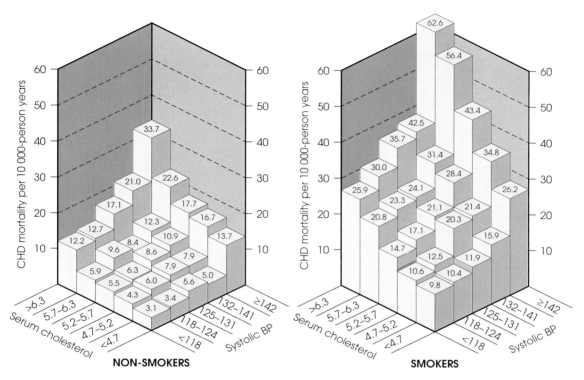

Figure 2.7

Coronary mortality rates in relation to smoking, blood pressure and cholesterol. Data from male examinees screened for the Multiple Risk Factor Intervention Trial (MRFIT).

hypertension, if left untreated, is around 12%. Patients with diastolic blood pressures between 130 and 150 mmHg but with no retinopathy have a 2-year survival rate of around 50% if left untreated (Fig. 2.5).

Moderate hypertensive patients with diastolic blood pressures between 110 and 129 mmHg have a 2-year survival rate of 80%. However, these statistics, the only ones available, are based on information obtained 40 years ago before the advent of effective antihypertensive drugs. Such patients now receive drug therapy and their mortality is correspondingly reduced, although not normalised.

With milder grades of hypertension, where diastolic blood pressures are between 95 and 105 mmHg, the annual mortality rate at the age of 45 years is about three times higher than in people whose pressures are nearer the average for the population. While this increased relative risk is marked, the absolute risk, that is, the chance of dying within 5 years, is fairly small, and many people with mild hypertension survive to a normal life expectancy.

Even people whose blood pressures are just above average for the population have an annual mortality at the age of 40 years of about 4 per 1000 so that, within 10 years,

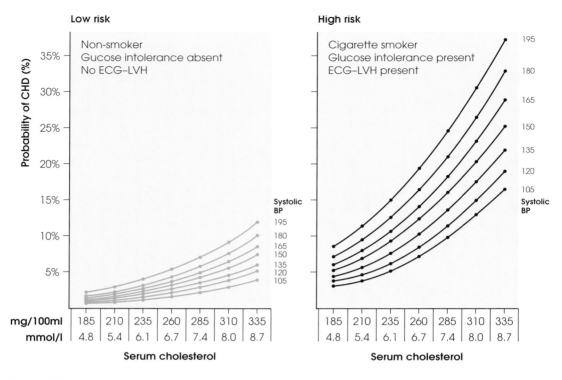

Figure 2.8
High and low risk of heart attacks. Data from the Framingham study.

4% will die of vascular disease attributable to hypertension. By contrast, people whose blood pressures are well below the population average have an annual mortality of about 3 per 1000.

In practical terms, the clinician should be aware that a man aged 35 years with a blood pressure of 150/100 mmHg has an odds-on chance of dying before he reaches the age of 60 years unless active steps are taken to reduce the pressure (Fig. 2.6). With advancing age, the risk of death for a given level of blood pressure increases. 'Clinical' hypertension roughly represents the top quintile of blood pressures of the population aged 45 years and carries a 3% annual death rate. The

same pressures at the age of 55 carry a 5% annual mortality, rising to 8% at the age of 65 years.

Multiple risk factors

As stated earlier, there are two other important and reversible cardiovascular risk factors in addition to raised blood pressure. These are cigarette smoking and raised blood lipids (Fig. 2.7). It is important to note that these three factors have a multiplicative or synergistic effect on each other. A person with two risk factors is much worse off than a person with only one. Thus a patient with mild

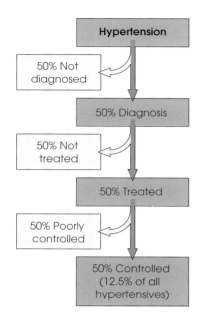

Figure 2.9
The rule of halves.

hypertension but no other risk factors is not at a particularly high risk compared with a similar patient who also smokes cigarettes and has an elevated plasma cholesterol.

When assessing the risk for an individual, all risk factors need to be taken into account, including concurrent glucose intolerance and the presence of LVH (Fig. 2.8). It is therefore important to estimate a patient's absolute risk of premature death. However, other factors that cannot be treated also influence survival rates and the chances of sustaining a heart attack or a stroke. Firstly, as stated earlier, age is an important consideration and, in general, the benefits of managing hypertension in the elderly are greater than in younger people. This is because they have a greater absolute risk of death, which is now known to be reversible

with drug therapy. Women have a lower risk than men at all levels of blood pressure up until the age of about 50 years when their risk steadily rises to the same level as seen in men. As discussed in more detail elsewhere, there are important ethnic differences in the risk of hypertension, with stroke being a particularly common problem among blacks, and coronary heart disease being a major cause of death among South Asians.

Another important factor that must be taken into account is the genetic influence, which exerts its effect independently of the three main cardiovascular risk factors. People with a family history of premature death, heart attack or stroke are at higher risk. This is only partly explained by familial similarities of lifestyle, diet and smoking habits.

There is now increasing evidence that a high salt intake and a low potassium intake as well as a high alcohol intake have adverse effects on stroke mortality rates, partially via raised blood pressure but also partly due to the direct effect on cerebral vasculature. By contrast, obesity, when it is not associated with hypertension, hyperlipidaemia or glucose intolerance, does not appear to be a major independent risk factor for cardiovascular death.

By any criteria, hypertension is important; it is also neglected. The main consideration in this chapter has been the risk of blood pressure to the individual as well as to the whole population. Most heart attacks and strokes occur in people whose pressures are either only mildly raised or are just above the average for the population. Although the individual's risk of death with near average blood pressure is small, the population attributable risk is high. This is because mild hypertension is very common, so the number of its vascular complications in the community is large. Primary care clinicians need to be concerned not only with blood pressures that are high enough to require antihypertensive drug therapy but also to see a lowering of blood pressures of all their patients. The goal of good medical care should include not only successful management of patients but also primary prevention, which can only be achieved with a well organised educational programme.

THE UNDERDIAGNOSIS OF HYPERTENSION

The term 'the rule of halves' was first coined in the early 1970s in the USA, and population studies in the UK, Europe and elsewhere have reported similar findings (Fig. 2.9). The rule of halves means that, unless special efforts are made, only half of all hypertensive people will be diagnosed. Furthermore, of those cases that are diagnosed, only about half will receive antihypertensive treatment and, of those, only half will have adequate control of their blood pressure. The end result is that only 10–15% of hypertensive patients receive adequate medical care, a situation that constitutes a national and international scandal. It has been calculated that in the UK around 300 people die from preventable hypertension-related disease every 6 weeks. If a fully laden jumbo jet were to crash every 6 weeks killing all its passengers the mortality figures would be about the same. If such an improbable series of disasters did occur, there would be a public outcry, while these hypertension-related deaths pass almost unnoticed.

Dangerous myths

The climate that has led to the 'rule of halves' is due in part to a series of dangerous myths and misconceptions. Doctors, health care administrators, politicians and patients are remarkably ignorant of the true priorities of medical care and the relative importance of chronic diseases like hypertension.

Myth 1

Cancer is the most important health hazard. Whilst cancer is seen as more terrifying and a more urgent medical problem, hypertension-related diseases kill more people than all other causes combined, including cancer, in men. Furthermore, hypertension is treatable and, therefore, premature deaths can be avoided. There is, however, scant evidence to show that medical care can favourably influence cancer mortality.

Myth 2

Severe hypertension is a more important hazard to health than mild hypertension. Although severe hypertension is a major cause of premature death, it is relatively rare. Mild hypertension with its lower risk, by contrast, is very common, and its prevention or cure could lead to a massive reduction in cardiovascular disease and premature death.

Myth 3

Hypertension is characterised by symptoms including headache and tiredness. In the past, practically all medical textbooks stated that hypertension causes headache, tiredness and other symptoms. More recent textbooks, however, draw attention to the fact that most people with hypertension are symptomless. There is only a very weak relationship between headache and epistaxis and the presence of mild to moderate hypertension. This means that hypertension cannot be relied upon to present with diagnostically useful symptoms at an early stage before development of the severe vascular complications of the disease.

Myth 4

Mild elevations of blood pressure are often due to some recent psychosocial stress and can be ignored. Single casual measurements of blood pressure during insurance medical examinations, for example, are very important predictors of risk. A man aged 35 with a single casual diastolic blood pressure of 100 mmHg or more is unlikely to survive until retirement age unless something is done to reduce his pressure. The prognosis of people with transiently elevated blood pressure is uncertain but they cannot be regarded as being without risk. They need careful follow-up. Recent evidence shows that patients with 'white coat' hypertension have a higher risk than those with persistently normal blood pressures.

Myth 5

Patients receiving drug therapy can stop once blood pressure is well controlled. Many patients hold the mistaken belief that antihypertensive drugs are, like antibiotics, only needed for a short course of treatment. This dangerous misconception is often the fault of the doctor, who has failed to explain the nature of the disease and its treatment to the patient. Very rarely and only under close supervision is it possible to stop therapy in patients with very mild hypertension. It is only feasible if pressures have been under excellent control for some years and where only a single antihypertensive drug has been necessary. Even then most patients are required to restart therapy over the ensuing years, and, anyway, all patients whose drug therapy has been discontinued need very active and careful follow-up.

Perhaps the biggest single reason for 'the rule of halves' is that the system of primary and secondary health care in most countries is not orientated towards the management of chronic diseases. It could be said that most countries have a national disease service rather than a national health service. Usually the doctor's role is rather like that of a shopkeeper. The patient presents with a symptom and is then given the appropriate treatment, frequently as a commercial transaction. The onus is on the patient to seek diagnosis, treatment and follow-up. The solution to 'the rule of halves' is to reverse the patient–doctor relationship so that the initiative is in the hands of health care professionals to seek out hypertensive patients and supervise the long-term control of their blood pressure and other risk factors. This is preventative medicine at its best.

Solutions

There are remarkably few diseases for which the mass screening of healthy populations can be justified. The main criteria for well population screening are:

* The disease must be sufficiently common to justify the efforts of examining millions of healthy people.
* The disease must be detectable at an early or presymptomatic stage.
* The disease must be worth treating at an early stage, contributing to prevention of death or disease.
* The screening technique should be cheap, simple and acceptable to healthy people.

- Screening and follow-up must be continuous, ongoing and feasible within the existing health care resources.

By all these criteria, hypertension is a suitable case for some form of screening. It affects up to 20% of the adult population, is easily detectable and is worth controlling. The main problem is the organisation of detection and follow-up programmes. Chapter 11 shows how this can be managed. This is one of the major contributions that the primary care team can make to the reduction of life-threatening levels of blood pressure in the population.

FURTHER READING

Lever AF, Harrap SB. Essential hypertension: a disorder of growth with origins in childhood? *J Hypertens* 1992; **10**: 101–20.

Hawthorne VM, Greaves DA, Beevers DG. Blood pressure in a Scottish town. *Br Med J* 1974; **3**: 600–3.

MacMahon S, Peto R, Cutler J, *et al*. Blood pressure, stroke, and coronary heart disease. Part 1, prolonged differences in blood pressure: prospective observational studies corrected for the regression dilution bias. *Lancet* 1990; **335**: 765–74.

Miall WE, Chinn S. Screening for hypertension: some epidemiological observations. *Br Med J* 1974; **3**: 595–600.

Nielsen WB, Vestlo J, Jensen GB. Isolated systolic hypertension as a major risk factor for stroke and myocardial infarction and an unexploited source of cardiovascular prevention: a prospective population-based study. *J Hum Hypertens* 1995; **9**: 175–80.

Poulter NR, Zographos D, Mattin R, *et al*, Concomitant risk factors in hypertensives: a survey of risk factors for cardiovascular disease amongst hypertensives in English general practices. *Blood Pressure* 1996; **5**: 209–15.

Smith WCS, Lee AJ, Crombie IK, Tunstall-Pedoe H. Control of blood pressure in Scotland: the rule of halves. *Br Med J* 1990; **300**: 981–3.

3 THE CAUSES OF HYPERTENSION: EPIDEMIOLOGICAL CLUES

BACKGROUND

The epidemiological view of hypertension differs from the clinical view. When considering national mortality and morbidity statistics, hypertension and hypertension-related deaths assume enormous proportions. This is mainly due to the very large numbers of mildly hypertensive people rather than the relatively small number with severe or malignant hypertension. The epidemiologists notice that the average blood pressure in all Western communities is a great deal higher than in rural African populations where hypertension and its vascular complications are almost unheard of. It is important, therefore, to work out why the average blood pressure of the whole population is raised and to investigate the many genetic and environmental factors that affect the blood pressure of the whole community.

Large surveys of population groups with accurate follow-up and notification of fatal and non-fatal cardiovascular events (cohort studies) are able to identify risk factors for hypertension and its related conditions. The object of this chapter is to discuss the information available from these surveys in relation to the cause of hypertension and also its prevention.

BLOOD PRESSURE AND AGE

Western countries

In Western countries, older people tend to have higher blood pressures than young people. Follow-up studies have demonstrated two important trends. Firstly, blood pressures rise with advancing age. Secondly, those individuals whose blood pressures start at a higher level tend to retain their place in the distribution of blood pressure and, also, sustain a faster age-related rise in pressure. This phenomenon of tracking is seen in all age groups, including infants (Fig. 3.1). It implies that whatever environmental factors influence blood pressure, they start to exert their effects at a very early age. This is not to deny that genetic factors have a role. It is probable that different populations and groups within populations do have genetically determined differences in susceptibility

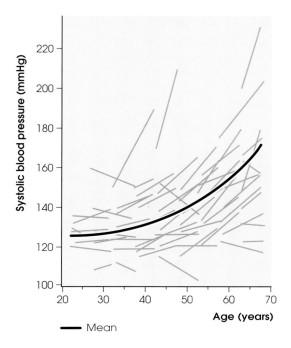

- Mean

Figure 3.1
Tracking of systolic blood pressure in a follow-up study in the population of Rhondda, South Wales. Initially and on rescreening a decade later.

to environmental influences. In Western societies it has been estimated that about 40% of the variation of blood pressure can be explained by genetic factors and about 40% by environmental factors. The remaining 20% are due to chance association and error.

The clear demonstration of a faster rise in blood pressure in people with higher than average pressures at early age also suggests that there may be some sort of 'vicious cycle' effect by which those individuals with higher pressures in early life tend to develop early structural changes in their arterioles, which in turn causes a further rise, particularly in systolic blood pressure. This rise then causes even more structural change and a further elevation of blood pressure.

Extreme old age

A slightly different picture emerges when examining the distribution of blood pressure in extremely old people (i.e. aged over age 85 years). Cross-sectional studies have shown that the average diastolic blood pressures of people at this age tend to be lower than those of people aged around 60 years. Longitudinal population surveys have also shown that elderly people genuinely do sustain a fall in diastolic pressure when they become very old, although their systolic blood pressures may continue to rise. This fall may not necessarily be physiological but is probably due to clinical or subclinical cardiac damage leading to a reduction of cardiac output. Other diseases associated with weight loss and general ill-health may also be present which may contribute to a lowering of blood pressure. Another possible factor is that those people who had raised blood pressures may have died earlier, leaving the survivors with lower pressures to take part in population surveys.

This selective mortality of hypertensive individuals may explain why over the age of about 85 there is an inverse relationship between the height of the blood pressure and the short-term mortality and morbidity from heart attacks and strokes; people with the lowest pressures having the highest mortality. This inverse relationship is probably explained by a blood pressure lowering effect of intercurrent cardiac disease or early

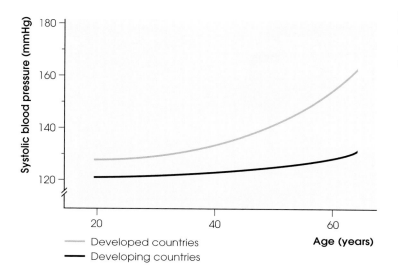

Figure 3.2
Changes in blood pressure in developed and developing countries.

cancer, causing premature death. More recently, well conducted follow-up studies of very old people have confirmed that the height of the blood pressure does accurately predict cardiovascular mortality in the longer term. This underlines the view that an individual's usual blood pressure is a potent cardiovascular risk factor at all ages.

Developing societies

Whatever the mechanisms that produce a rise in blood pressure with age, there is no reason to suppose that they are physiological. Studies of non-Westernised rural populations have shown that hypertension is unknown in these groups, and blood pressures show only a tiny rise with advancing age (Fig. 3.2). By contrast, in genetically similar people and even relatives living in urban communities, particularly in Africa, a marked rise in blood pressure is seen with age. A recent detailed migration study from

Kenya has shown that tribesmen whose pressures are initially low when seen in rural areas sustain a rapid rise in blood pressure within months of migration to Nairobi. Thus, the rise in blood pressure seen with advancing age in urban societies must be due primarily to some very powerful environmental factors. The likely factors are differences in diet and other socio-economic factors, including environmental stress. However, these influences may have more marked effects in people with some genetic predisposition to develop hypertension in the first place.

BLOOD PRESSURE AND GENETICS

Family history

High blood pressure tends to run in families (Fig. 3.3). Furthermore, the 'normotensive'

31

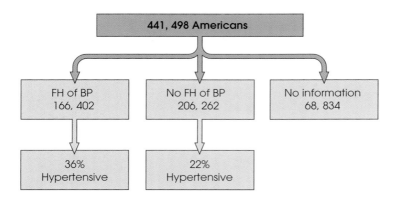

Figure 3.3
Hypertension in relation to family history.

children of hypertensive patients tend to have higher blood pressures than age-matched children of people with normal blood pressures. This familial concordance of blood pressure may, in part, be due to shared exposure to environmental influences, including diet and stress, but there does remain a large genetic component. This is well demonstrated by studies of monozygotic and dizygotic twins who were brought up separately and together, as well as studies of adopted and non-adopted children, their siblings and their parents (Fig. 3.4).

Genetic susceptibility

The genetic component of the development of high blood pressure may not itself necessarily cause hypertension. Rather, there may be a genetic predisposition to develop raised pressure in response to various environmental factors. There is some suggestion, although the data are not impressive, that normotensive offspring of hypertensive parents may be more susceptible to the pressor effects of high salt intake, environmental noise, isometric exercise, mental arithmetic and even high alcohol intake.

It is possible that the cause of the rise in blood pressure with age and thus the cause of hypertension may be found by investigating children, babies or even neonates. Again it is important to ascertain those influences that are genetic and those that are due to poor social environment. For instance, several studies by Professor David Barker have shown that babies with a relatively low birth weight (excluding those with intrauterine growth retardation) have a higher prevalence of hypertension in later life. This low birth weight may be thought to be related to poor socio-economic and environmental conditions experienced by their mothers during pregnancy. However, it now appears that babies with relatively low birth weights were born to mothers with blood pressures in the upper part of the normal distribution. Their tendency to develop higher pressures in adult life may therefore be more closely related to genetic factors.

RACE AND BLOOD PRESSURE

Clues into the aetiology of hypertension may also be obtained from comparison of differ-

Systolic blood pressure

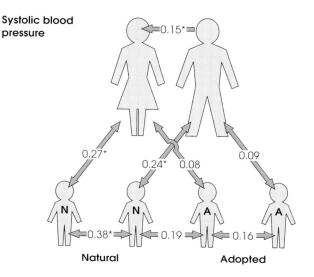

Natural   **Adopted**

Figure 3.4

Correlation coefficients of systolic and diastolic blood pressures between parents and their natural and adopted children in the Montreal adoption study. (*Clin Exp Hypertens* 1986; **8**: 653–60.)

Diastolic blood pressure

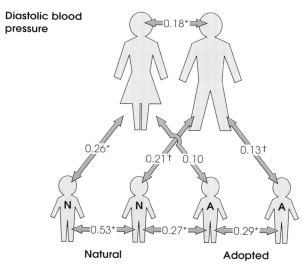

Natural   **Adopted**

*Significant at the 0.001 level of probability

†Significant at the 0.01 level of probability

ent racial groups. Most studies of blood pressure in black and white people in the UK and the USA have reported a higher average blood pressure in blacks and, consequently, a higher prevalence of hyper-

tension. Hypertension is also common in urban Africa. By contrast, blacks living in rural Africa have low blood pressures and no rise with advancing age. The Kenya Luo migration study demonstrated that the

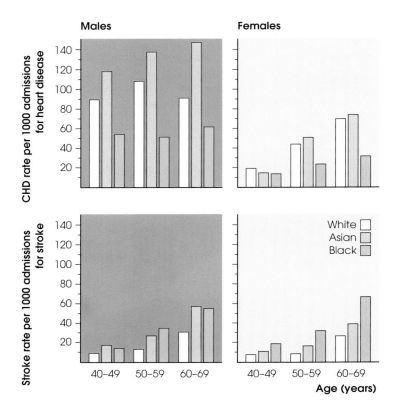

Figure 3.5
Coronary Heart Disease (CHD) and strokes in blacks, whites and Asians. Data on hospital admissions in Birmingham, UK.

marked rise in blood pressure with urbanisation occurred in association with a sharp rise in sodium intake and a fall in potassium intake. It has been suggested that in the hunter–gatherer societies of rural Africa thousands of years ago, a genetically determined tendency to retain the relatively small amount of salt in the diet conveyed a biological advantage. This tendency, however, became a disadvantage in urbanised societies where salt intake, often from junk food, is high.

Within Westernised countries, however, the higher blood pressures in black people are still apparent after correction for socio-economic and dietary factors as well as obesity. While in the UK and the USA, blacks are more likely to be unemployed, poor or stressed and may also receive inferior medical care, there is every reason to believe that, in part, hypertension is due to some racially determined factors. Most clinicians are aware that hypertension seems to be rather different in blacks with differences in responses to antihypertensive drugs. Black hypertensive patients are less sensitive to beta-blockers and angiotensin-converting enzyme (ACE) inhibitors. They also have lower plasma renin and angiotensin levels.

While hypertension is definitely more common in black people in the USA and UK, they have less coronary heart disease than white people but considerably more strokes (Fig. 3.5). It remains uncertain, however, whether, for a given level of blood pressure, blacks have a higher risk of death than white people. Most population surveys have shown that black people have lower serum total cholesterol levels and higher HDL cholesterol levels than whites. This may, in part, explain their apparent protection from coronary heart disease. However, it is probable that the differences in coronary heart disease between blacks and whites cannot be entirely explained by differences in the three known coronary risk factors, hypertension, cigarette smoking and hyperlipidaemia. A higher prevalence of glucose intolerance in blacks (and also South Asians) may be one explanation, and there are important ethnic differences in plasma fibrinogen levels.

Other ethnic groups

There are few reliable studies of other ethnic minority groups in Western countries. Hypertension is known to be common among people of Indian and Pakistani origin in the UK and Trinidad. The relatively small number of studies conducted in the Indian subcontinent suggest the rise in blood pressure with advancing age is more evident in urban than in rural populations. Asians in the UK have higher rates of coronary heart disease than whites, even though their blood pressures are not higher.

There is considerably more information about hypertension amongst Japanese people. In Japan, high blood pressure is very common and, in line with this, the incidence of stroke is also very high. By contrast, coronary heart disease is rare in Japan. Comparisons with Japanese migrants to Honolulu and the west coast of the USA have shown that, with increasing adoption of American lifestyles and diet, there is a reduction in hypertension and stroke incidence but a marked rise in coronary heart disease. These studies, therefore, confirm a very powerful effect of environmental factors on hypertension and its complications.

BLOOD PRESSURE AND GENDER

Below the age of about 45, women tend to have slightly lower blood pressures than men. They also have less coronary heart disease and strokes. These differences in early life may be due to endocrinological events associated with the childbearing years (Fig. 3.6). High blood pressure remains a risk factor for

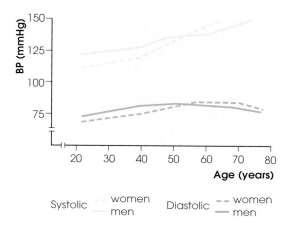

Figure 3.6

Changes in blood pressure with age in men and women.

heart attacks and strokes in premenopausal women but the gradient of blood pressure and risk is less steep than in men.

Blood pressure and pregnancy

There is a weak tendency for women who have had hypertension in pregnancy to develop high blood pressure in later life. The topic of hypertension in pregnancy is covered in more detail in Chapter 16.

Blood pressure and the menopause

After the age of about 50 years, blood pressures rise in women to become similar to those seen in men. At the same time, heart attack and stroke rates increase. The relative absence of hypertension and cardiovascular disease in women before the menopause raised the possibility that endogenous oestrogens are in some way protective. However, high doses of synthetic oestrogens as are used in the oral contraceptive pill certainly confer no benefit and occasionally themselves cause hypertension. In postmenopausal women who have low endogenous oestrogen levels, replacement with low-dose natural oestrogens does not appear to cause any rise in blood pressure and may be protective against coronary heart disease (see also Chapter 14).

The gradient of blood pressure and cardiovascular events in post-menopausal women is similar to that in men but is said to be delayed by about 10 years. Thus a woman aged 60 years has about the same risk as a man aged 50 years.

SOCIOLOGICAL AND DIETARY FACTORS

Weight

Fat people have higher blood pressures than thin people (Fig. 3.7). There is, however, an important confounding factor to be taken into account. There is a tendency to overestimate blood pressure in people with fat arms particularly if the blood pressure cuffs are too small. The fatter the arm, the greater the overestimation. However, after correction for arm circumference, there still remains a positive relationship between body mass index (BMI) and both systolic and diastolic blood pressure. Recent statistical analysis suggests that BMI exerts its effects mainly on diastolic blood pressure with little independent effect on the systolic pressure, which is mainly related to age.

The mechanism by which obese people have a high blood pressure is uncertain. It is probable that obese people eat more sodium and less potassium and, therefore, may develop a rise in blood pressure due to dietary factors. It is probable also that high blood pressure is more closely correlated with central obesity than with BMI alone. More recently, intravenous glucose tolerance tests have demonstrated that obese people are relatively resistant to insulin, and this concept is now the subject of a great deal of research. It has been postulated that insulin resistance leads to a rise in intracellular sodium concentration and to renal retention of salt and water. Thus, insulin itself may play some role in the aetiology of essential hypertension, particularly in obese individuals.

Since obesity is itself associated with high blood lipid levels, glucose intolerance and high blood pressure, fat people are more prone to coronary heart disease. It is possible, however, that after allowing for these factors, BMI alone may not itself be an independent cardiovascular risk factor. This is only a theoretical consideration as most obese people do have the other cardiovascular risk factors and thus have a high risk of death. When people lose weight, their blood pressures tend to fall at a rate of 1 mm Hg/kg reduction of body weight.

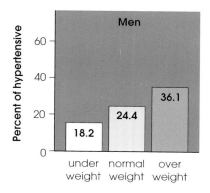

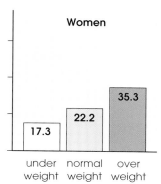

Figure 3.7

The relationship between obesity and high blood pressures (From Stamler, R, et al.)

Salt

The first suggestion that a high salt intake gives rise to high blood pressure goes back 4000 years to the ancient Chinese Yellow Emperor, Huang Ti. He suggested that people who ate too much salt developed harder pulses. More recent epidemiological evidence is so impressive that the salt hypothesis can no longer be considered controversial.

As stated earlier, primitive rural societies in Africa and also the South Pacific islands consume very little salt (below 50 mmol/day) and have hardly any hypertension and no rise in blood pressure with age. Conversely, European, American and Japanese populations consume a lot of salt (200–300 mmol/day) and have high average blood pressures. The very high incidence of strokes amongst the northern Japanese may well be related to their very high salt intake, and the recent impressive reduction in stroke rates may well be attributable to the reduction in salt intake that has occurred over the last 20 years.

The INTERSALT project was a major international collaborative study in which directly comparable data were obtained from 52

different populations in 32 countries. All the important confounding differences between urban or Westernised populations and primitive groups were taken into account. The study showed unequivocally that the rise in blood pressure seen with advancing age in urban but not rural populations was related to the amount of salt in the diet (Fig. 3.8). Similarly, a recent overview or meta-analysis of all the reliable individual population surveys of blood pressure in relation to salt intake confirmed the close relationship between salt intake and the height of the blood pressure, and demonstrated that this effect was independent of the degree of urbanisation.

There is evidence that over the last 50 years, dietary salt consumption in the USA and Europe has fallen, and this has been paralleled by a fall in stroke incidence. The fall in stroke incidence since the Second World War is only partly due to the more frequent use of antihypertensive medication. Also, there is now evidence that high salt intake may cause strokes, partly through a direct effect on cerebral vessels and partly by a concomitant high prevalence of hypertension.

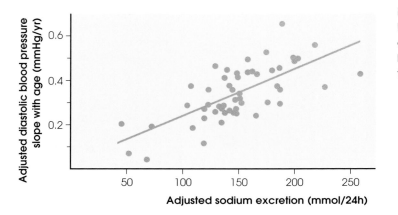

Figure 3.8
Relationship between sodium excretion and the rise of blood pressure with age. Data from the INTERSALT project.

It used to be said that while international comparisons support the salt story, individual national studies do not. However, in the INTERSALT project, a positive relationship was found between salt intake and systolic blood pressure in 39 of the 52 populations examined, and this association was statistically significant in 15 populations.

The salt hypothesis receives further confirmation from observations that extreme salt loading can cause a rise in blood pressure and that modest salt restriction causes a significant fall in blood pressure in both hypertensive and normotensive people.

Taking all these facts into account, it is our opinion that the salt hypothesis should no longer be regarded as a controversial hypothesis, but more as a confirmed mechanism.

Potassium

The role of potassium in lowering blood pressure has received less attention until recently. International comparisons of blood pressure and potassium intake, and notably the INTERSALT project, have shown that a higher potassium intake appears to be associated with a lower prevalence of hypertension. It is also probable that a low potassium intake has an independent effect on stroke mortality, which is separate from the effect of blood pressure. Sodium and potassium cannot easily be considered separately, and when assessing their effects, it is probably best to examine dietary or urinary sodium/potassium ratios.

It is interesting to note that in the USA, where hypertension is common in blacks, there are virtually no differences in sodium intake or urinary sodium excretion between blacks and whites but there are marked differences in potassium intake and excretion. Black people tend to consume lower quantities of potassium-rich foods, which are usually of high quality and expensive. This may explain partly some of the social and economic factors causing racial differences in blood pressure.

Alcohol

Most epidemiological studies have shown a close positive relationship between alcohol

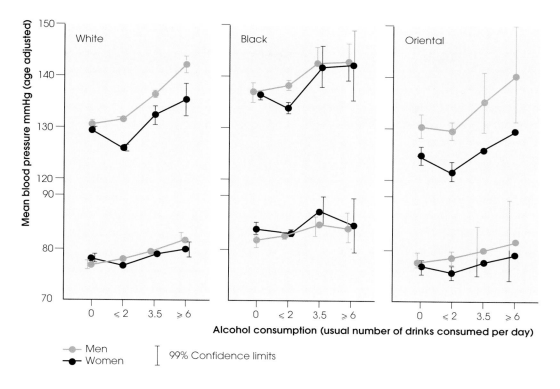

Figure 3.9

Relationship between alcohol intake and blood pressure. Data from Kaiser Permanente Health Insurance Program.

consumption and blood pressure. This was evident in the INTERSALT project. There is also evidence for a correlation between a high alcohol intake and stroke mortality and morbidity in both community and clinical studies. There is a trend, however, for the lowest blood pressures to be recorded in those people who regularly consume small amounts of alcohol when compared with people who drink no alcohol at all. Strangely, 'teetotallers' seem to have slightly higher blood pressures than moderate

drinkers (Fig. 3.9). This is probably due to the fact that some people who claim that they do not drink have, in fact, stopped drinking for medical reasons or they may have deceived their enquirers. Alternatively, teetotallers may genuinely have slightly higher blood pressures. This would imply that small amounts of alcohol lower blood pressure but large amounts of alcohol raise it.

In heavy drinkers, hypertension is common, and the more they drink, the higher their blood pressures are. Hypertensive patients have a higher frequency of raised liver enzymes (gamma glutamyltransferase) and higher mean erythrocyte cell volumes (MCV). It has been estimated that about 10% of hypertensive people have alcohol-induced hypertension.

Several reliable clinical studies have demonstrated that a reduction of alcohol intake causes a significant fall in blood pressure. In view of the reversibility of alcohol-associated high blood pressure, it is important that clinicians attempt to moderate the amount of alcohol their patients consume, where possible avoiding antihypertensive drugs.

The mechanism by which alcohol raises blood pressure remains unknown. It is possible that amongst very heavy drinkers, the height of the blood pressure is more closely related to the symptoms and signs of alcohol withdrawal rather than to the alcohol itself. During alcohol withdrawal, many patients develop sympathetic overactivity, and very high plasma noradrenaline levels have been reported.

In contrast, acute alcohol loading studies conducted amongst hypertensive and normotensive volunteers have shown that alcohol causes a rapid rise in blood pressure and a rapid fall afterwards, and that this relationship closely follows the blood alcohol levels. This acute rise in blood pressure in response to alcohol may be due to the direct effect of alcohol on vascular smooth muscle.

Population surveys also tend to support a relatively acute affect of alcohol on blood pressure. Examinees in such surveys who have drunk heavily in the days prior to screening tend to have higher blood pressures. By contrast, people who drank heavily more than 3 days before being examined but have drunk nothing in the 3 days immediately prior to screening have lower blood pressures.

These findings have led to the hypothesis that alcohol does not so much cause hypertension but causes transient elevations in blood pressure, which are detectable in clinical practice and lead to the individual being labelled as hypertensive. This paradox may explain why there is no convincing evidence that a high alcohol intake is associated with coronary heart disease, except possibly amongst binge drinkers, who may have an increased risk of arrhythmic death following a heart attack. Possibly, however, the effects of alcohol on blood pressure are offset by a beneficial effect on HDL cholesterol.

Coffee and blood pressure

A great many studies have shown that there is a positive link between coffee consumption and coronary heart disease. This may be partly explained by the confounding effect of concomitant cigarette smoking and a high-cholesterol diet. There is also some evidence that coffee consumption causes an acute but reversible rise in blood pressure. Recently, a long-term study has shown that continued abstinence from coffee over a period of several weeks may slightly reduce blood pressure.

Animal fats

In general, vegetarians have lower blood pressures than non-vegetarians but it is uncertain why this difference occurs. After correction for the effects of the associated salt content of non-vegetarian meals, this effect seems to persist. This has led to the hypothesis that a high animal fat diet itself may be related to hypertension. It is possible also that the high fibre content of a vegetarian diet may explain its protective action against hypertension. There is, however, also some evidence that the consumption of a high-protein diet may protect against hypertension.

Calcium

Some population studies have reported a positive correlation between blood pressure and serum total calcium concentrations. There is, however, little convincing evidence that high blood pressure is related to either a low or a high calcium intake in the diet. It has been suggested that a low-calcium diet may contribute to raised blood pressure in some populations, but these data remain controversial. More recently, an overview of all the studies of calcium loading has shown that this manoeuvre has a negligible effect on blood pressure.

Smoking

After one or two cigarettes have been smoked, blood pressure may rise sharply. Despite this acute effect, epidemiological studies have shown no relationship or even a negative correlation between blood pressure and cigarette smoking. Non-smokers have a slightly higher blood pressure than smokers, and people who stop smoking sometimes sustain a small rise in blood pressure. These differences may be due to changes in body weight. Heavy smokers are thinner, iller and more breathless, and when they stop smoking, they eat more and gain weight. Although smoking is not related closely to blood pressure, it is of course a potent independent risk factor for both heart attack and stroke. Hypertensive patients who are also smokers have a much higher risk of death for a given level of blood pressure.

There is one rare but interesting exception to the rule that cigarette smoking and blood pressure are negatively associated. Several studies have shown that the prevalence of cigarette smoking is high amongst malignant hypertensive people compared with non-malignant hypertensives and the general population. Cigarette smoking is also closely associated with atheromatous renal artery stenosis.

Blood pressures and social class

In Western countries, blood pressures as well as coronary heart disease and stroke rates tend to be lower in people from higher social classes. It is probable that these differences can be explained by differences in smoking, salt intake, alcohol consumption and BMI. More recently, it has been suggested that intrauterine undernutrition, which is also related to poverty, may be a factor in the aetiology of hypertension in later life. It remains uncertain, however, whether the social class differences in blood pressure can all be explained on the basis of other concomitant environmental factors.

In the USA, it has been demonstrated that the highest social class blacks still have higher blood pressures than the lowest social class whites (Fig. 3.10). It is important to note that in the developing countries of Africa, the social class/hypertension relationship is the reverse of that seen in Europe. Strokes and hypertension are commoner in people who are in the executive and managerial classes in West Africa, and these are the most economically active. The situation in Africa now resembles that seen in the UK before

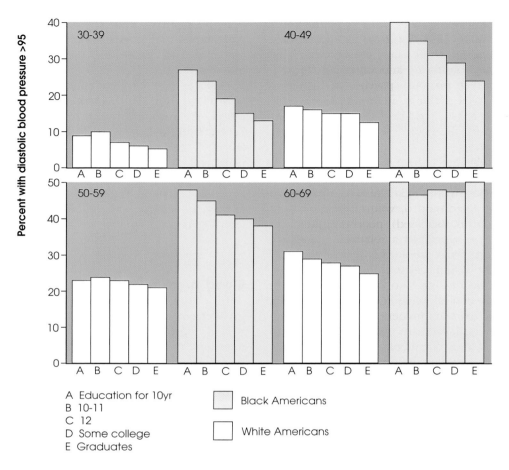

Figure 3.10

Hypertension in relation to the duration of education in black and white Americans.

the 1939–45 war. Nutritional factors must explain these trends and this will be the basis of a new major international study, (INTERMAP), which was established in 1996.

Stress

As hypertension is a disease of Westernised, and particularly of urban, societies (although large urban/rural differences are not seen much in Europe and the USA), it is tempting to attribute high blood pressure to the stress of modern living. Certainly, acutely stressful stimuli raise blood pressure and may be more pressor in subjects who have hypertension. However, there remains considerable doubt as to whether chronic stress raises blood pressure. Investigation of environmental stress and high blood pressure in population surveys is confounded by other social factors, including poverty, dietary fats, calorie, electrolyte and alcohol intake and cigarette smoking. Studies of various psychosocial indices, including aggression, neuroticism and introversion, have produced conflicting results. Many reliable studies have found no clear-cut effects.

In individuals, there is some evidence of a relationship between stress and hypertension. The type A/type B classification of personality has demonstrated, with many exceptions, that type A (stressed) people have higher blood pressures and a relatively higher risk of death than type B people. However, hypertensive patients may only develop higher stress levels once they have been diagnosed and made to worry about their health. The term 'hypertensive personality' is misleading and may only be an accurate description of people who are called frequently to attend the blood pressure clinic.

Exercise

Dynamic exercise raises blood pressure and isometric exercise raises it a lot. Despite this, there is good evidence that people who take regular exercise are healthier and have lower blood pressures than those who take none. There is evidence that regular exercise decreases coronary heart disease in normotensive and hypertensive people (Fig. 3.11). This may be partly because they are thinner and tend to have more sensible dietary, drinking and smoking habits.

More recently, a study of the effects of different levels of exercise in a randomised controlled trial have demonstrated that increasing exercise lowers blood pressure independently from any other dietary manoeuvres.

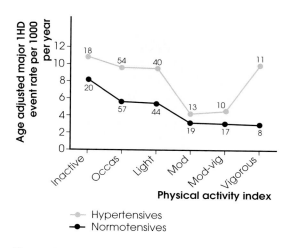

Figure 3.11
Exercise and coronary heart disease. Data from the British Regional Heart Study.

Trace metals

It has been claimed that both cadmium and lead, which are environmental pollutants, may cause high blood pressure. Many of these associations have not been confirmed by detailed studies that have taken concurrent alcohol intake into account. The main source of cadmium to the human body is cigarette smoke. The evidence for the trace metal hypertension hypothesis must now be regarded as very fragile, although a positive correlation between blood lead and blood pressure does appear to be genuine even after correction for possible confounding variables. Conversely, however, there is fairly good evidence that blood pressures are lower in areas where the drinking water is hard (i.e. has a higher calcium content), although the mechanisms for this association are unknown.

Ambient temperature

There is a fairly close relationship between blood pressure and ambient temperature. In the northern hemisphere, blood pressures settle in the summer when it is warmer. There is less variation in blood pressure in areas where there is less seasonal variation in temperature. In the UK, blood pressures tend to be higher in the winter and, similarly, stroke mortality is also high at this time. This may be due to a direct pressor effect of cold weather. Conversely, in warm weather people may be more cheerful and relaxed, they may lose more sodium in sweat and may be relatively vasodilated. This effect of ambient temperature on blood pressure is of little clinical importance but is an important confounding variable to be taken into account in population surveys.

CONCLUSIONS

The epidemiologist's view of hypertension has led to the identification of a series of risk factors that are relevant to clinical practice. It is also true that reversal of these environmental factors in populations could have a greater impact on mortality and morbidity from hypertension-related disease than only the efficient care of those individuals with high pressures.

Even after taking into account all the environmental and genetic influences discussed in this chapter, a large amount of variation of blood pressure between populations remains unexplained. For this reason, epidemiological research must be continued and novel possible risk factors need to be investigated.

FURTHER READING

Boshuizen HC, Izaks GJ, von Buuren S, *et al.* Blood pressure and mortality in elderly people aged 85 and over: community based study. *Br Med J* 1998; **316**: 1780–4.

Elliott P, Stamler J, Nichols R, *et al.* For the Intersalt Cooperative Research Group. Intersalt revisited: further analyses of 24 hour sodium excretion and blood pressure within and across populations. *Br Med J* 1996; **312**: 1249–53.

Havlik RJ, Feinleib M. Epidemiology and genetics of hypertension. *Hypertension* 1982; **4** (Suppl 3): 121–7.

HDFP Co-operative Group. Race, education and prevalence of hypertension. *Am J Epidiol* 1977; **106**: 351–61.

Klatsky A, Friedman GD, Siegelaub MS, *et al.* Alcohol consumption and blood pressure. Kaiser–Permanente multiphasic health examination data. *N Engl J Med* 1977; **296**: 1194–200.

Mongeau J-G, Bion P, Sing CF. The influence of genetics and household environment upon the variability of blood pressure: the Montreal adoption study. *Clin Exp Hypertens* 1986; **8**: 653–60.

Perry IJ, Whincup PH, Shapter AG. Environmental factors in the development of essential hypertension. *Br Med Bull* 1994; **50**: 246–59.

Staessen J, Bulpitt CJ, Fagard R, *et al.* The influence of menopause on blood pressure. *J Hum Hypertens* 1989; **3**: 427–33.

Stamler R, Stamler J, Riedlinger, *et al.* Weight and blood pressure. Findings in hypertension screening of 1 million Americans. *JAMA* 1978; **240**: 1607–10.

Stamler R, Stamler J, Riedlinger WF, *et al.* Family (parental) history and prevalence of hypertension. *JAMA* 1979; **241**: 43–6.

Whelton PK, Epidemiology of hypertension. *Lancet* 1994; **344**: 101–6.

4 FACTORS CONTROLLING BLOOD PRESSURE

BACKGROUND

This chapter discusses the mechanisms known to control blood pressure in normal people and those factors that may raise it both in patients with essential hypertension and in the small minority of patients with an underlying cause of their raised pressures. Studies in the community and also in general practice have shown that less than 2% of patients with high blood pressure have an identifiable underlying cause. Even in hospital practice, less than 10% of cases have a renal or adrenal disease underlying their hypertension. Hence, in the majority of people with raised blood pressure the cause is not known. Rather than call this 'hypertension of unknown cause' it is usually labelled 'primary hypertension' or, more commonly, 'essential hypertension'. A great deal of research has been centred on the mechanisms underlying essential hypertension. An understanding of these mechanisms might help prevent the development of high blood pressure. This is preferable to having to treat blood pressure at a relatively late stage in the course of the disease.

MECHANISMS FOR MAINTAINING NORMAL BLOOD PRESSURE

The height of the blood pressure is determined by the amount of blood that is pumped out by the heart and by the resistance to flow in the peripheral arterial tree. The major resistance to flow is not in the large arteries or the capillaries but in the small arterioles. These arterioles are highly contractile and at all times constricted to some degree. The degree of constriction for a given cardiac output determines the height of the blood pressure. Variations in this degree of constriction from one area to another also regulate regional blood flow.

There are many complex systems regulating the degree of resistance in the arterioles as well as cardiac output. For example, during exercise there is an increase in cardiac output but a large reduction in peripheral vascular resistance in the arterioles supplying the voluntary muscles. Blood pressure therefore tends to remain relatively constant.

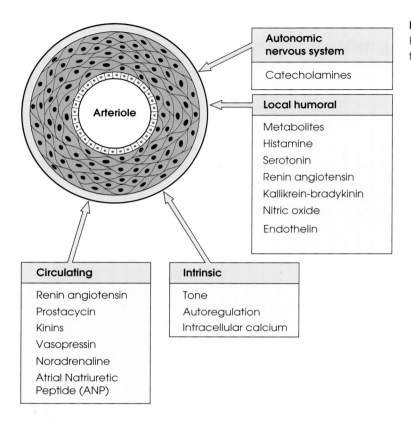

Figure 4.1
Factors affecting arteriolar tone.

Cardiac output

In patients with established hypertension, cardiac output is normal, and the elevated blood pressure is due to a raised peripheral vascular resistance. In very severe hypertension when the heart is under strain, cardiac output may fall and left ventricular failure may supervene, particularly where there is associated coronary artery disease. It has been suggested that in the early phase of the development of essential hypertension, cardiac output is raised and peripheral resistance is normal, and that, as blood pressure rises over the ensuing years, peripheral resistance rises and cardiac output returns to normal. However, evidence for this is not convincing. Subjects studied are likely to be more anxious and, thereby, have increased cardiac output when first examined.

Left ventricular hypertrophy

Due to the increased resistance to blood flow, the left ventricle has to pump harder and enlarges. This maintains cardiac output but in the longer term may lead to heart failure and an increased incidence of cardiac arrhythmias. For a given level of blood pressure, the cardiovascular mortality is three to four times higher if there is concomitant left ventricular hypertrophy (LVH) on ECG or echocardiology. It is possible also that LVH may develop independently of blood pressure. Those factors that cause peripheral vasoconstriction may also promote the thickening of the wall of the ventricle. Thus, LVH may not, like heart attack and stroke, simply be a consequence of hypertension.

Peripheral resistance

The walls of the small arterioles contain smooth muscle cells that respond to both local and circulating hormonal influences and to neural input through the autonomic nervous system. The degree of contraction of smooth muscle cells is thought to be determined by their intracellular free calcium content. Calcium is normally found in very low concentrations in cells compared with plasma, so in order to maintain this gradient, calcium pumps on the cell membrane extrude calcium from the cell to the outside. There are also mechanisms within the cell controlling intracellular calcium. Several lines of evidence now suggest that the increased tone in the arteriolar smooth muscle cells in patients with high blood pressure may be related to an increase in calcium in these cells.

There is also evidence that increased pressure within the arterioles leads to the development of structural changes within the vessels. The vessels become thicker, so that the internal lumen is further reduced, and this may lead to a further increase in peripheral resistance and blood pressure. This vascular hypertrophy or remodelling may possibly be independent of the rise in blood pressure and may be due to vascular growth factors either generated within the

arteriolar smooth muscle, the endothelium, or from the circulation.

Regulation of peripheral resistance

The degree of constriction of the arterioles is controlled by many factors (Fig. 4.1). Nearly all arterioles have the intrinsic ability to regulate flow, so that if it is increased the arterioles constrict to reduce flow, and if it is reduced the arterioles dilate. This so-called 'autoregulation' may be dependent on local metabolites, although increasing evidence suggests that it may also be related to local hormones released by the endothelium. One of the most important is nitric oxide, previously known as endothelial derived relaxant factor, and its relationship with the powerful vasoconstrictor, endothelin.

The autonomic nervous system

The autonomic nervous system, particularly the sympathetic system, can cause both constriction and dilation of arteriolar smooth muscle. Under normal circumstances, the circulating amounts of noradrenaline (norepinephrine) and adrenaline (epinephrine) play only a small role in determining the degree of constriction of arterioles. Most circulating noradrenaline is derived from spill-over from peripheral sympathetic ganglia or nerve endings where it is a major neurotransmitter; relatively little is derived from secretion by the adrenal gland. The major effect of the sympathetic nervous system on the arterioles is through the nerves that directly supply them. Drugs that block the sympathetic system, including the alpha- and beta-blockers, lower blood pressure in both normotensive and hypertensive subjects, clearly illustrating the important role that the autonomic nervous system has in maintaining peripheral resistance, and thereby blood pressure, in both hypertensive and normotensive subjects.

Overactivity of the sympathetic nervous system has been suggested as a possible cause of essential hypertension. Early papers appeared to show a relationship between plasma noradrenaline levels and blood pressure, although these did not take into account the rise in plasma noradrenaline levels with advancing age. Furthermore, assessing the activity of the sympathetic nervous system is extremely difficult. Plasma levels of noradrenaline and adrenaline reflect sympathetic activity rather poorly and, in particular, do not reflect regional differences in sympathetic outflow. Therefore, at present, there is little evidence that increased sympathetic activity causes high blood pressure. On the other hand, the sympathetic nervous system has a very important role in the short-term variations in blood pressure, particularly in response to stress, exercise and changes in posture.

The renin–angiotensin–aldosterone system

The renin–angiotensin–aldosterone system, like the sympathetic nervous system, is an important mechanism that maintains normal blood pressure, and both systems are closely integrated. The various components of the renin system can readily be measured, and therefore assessment of the activity of the system is easier than that of the sympathetic nervous system. Renin is an enzyme secreted by the juxtaglomerular cells in the cortex of the kidney. In the plasma it cleaves off a small peptide, angiotensin I, from a large circulating protein (renin substrate or angiotensinogen), which is made in the liver. Angiotensin I has no physiological action but is immediately converted to the octapeptide angiotensin II by angiotensin-converting enzyme (ACE).

Angiotensin II is one of the most potent vasoconstrictors known, causing contraction of both the small arterioles and veins. It can also stimulate the sympathetic nervous system by a direct effect on the brain and indirectly by increasing peripheral neurotransmission. It is also an important stimulus for the secretion of aldosterone from the adrenal gland. Both aldosterone and angiotensin II itself cause the kidney to retain sodium. The activity of the renin–angiotensin system is closely related to concurrent dietary salt intake; as more salt is consumed, the amount of circulating angiotensin II decreases. If salt intake is reduced there is a large rise in renin and angiotensin II levels. Other stimuli for the release of renin are the sympathetic nervous system and the baroreceptors in the renal arterioles, which directly respond to a fall in pressure by increasing renin release.

Various inhibitors of the renin system have been developed (Fig 4.2). Beta-blockers cause a fall in renin release by about 50%. There are also direct renin inhibitors but as yet the only oral one available is short-acting and poorly absorbed. More important are the ACE inhibitors, which directly block the enzyme that converts angiotensin I to angiotensin II. They are widely used in the treatment of high blood pressure and heart failure. Recently, direct orally absorbed competitive antagonists of angiotensin II for its receptor site have been developed, and have become another major way of blocking the system. Studies with these different inhibitors have clearly shown that the renin–angiotensin system is an important buffer system that regulates blood

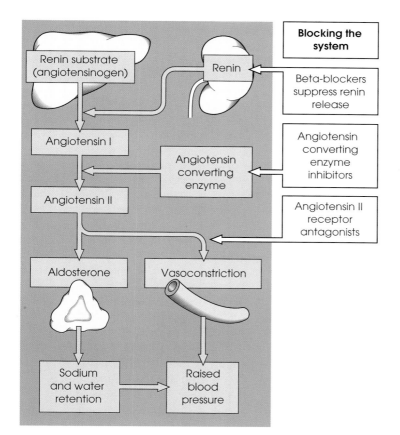

Blocking the system

Beta-blockers suppress renin release

Angiotensin converting enzyme inhibitors

Angiotensin II receptor antagonists

Figure 4.2
The renin–angiotensin system and site of action of drugs that block the system.

pressure under normal conditions and tries to maintain blood pressure under different volume conditions at the same level (e.g. alteration of salt intake).

In view of the important role of the renin system in regulating normal blood pressure, it is not surprising that it also plays an important role in regulating blood pressure in essential hypertension. However, whether it is involved in the cause of high blood pressure is much more debatable. In general, patients with essential hypertension have lower circulating levels of renin and angiotensin II than normotensive individuals of the same age. Only in renovascular hypertension, where the renal artery is narrowed and the perfusion pressure of the glomeruli is reduced, and in malignant or accelerated hypertension, where there is direct damage to the afferent arterioles, again leading to a fall in glomerular pressure, are large amounts of renin secreted. In these few patients, the raised levels of angiotensin II are the immediate direct cause of the high blood pressure.

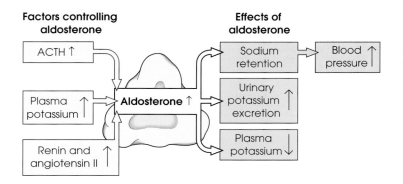

Factors controlling aldosterone

Effects of aldosterone

Figure 4.3

Factors controlling aldosterone release and its systemic effects.

Aldosterone is a potent sodium-retaining mineralocorticoid hormone secreted by the adrenal cortex. Its main action is on the distal renal tubules, increasing the exchange of sodium for potassium, thereby causing sodium retention at the expense of potassium loss (Fig. 4.3). In man, aldosterone release is mainly under the control of angiotensin II.

Atrial natriuretic peptide

The atria of the heart secrete peptides that play an important role in regulating sodium balance by a direct effect of increasing sodium excretion from the renal tubules as well as indirectly by suppressing renin release (Fig. 4.4). Plasma levels of atrial natriuretic peptides are raised in many patients with essential hypertension. Drugs that block the breakdown of atrial natriuretic peptides have been developed; these atriopeptidase inhibitors raise the endogenous levels of atrial peptides two-to-threefold. The drugs developed so far are not very effective in lowering blood pressure unless they are combined with an ACE inhibitor.

Vasopressin

Vasopressin (antidiuretic hormone) is secreted by the posterior pituitary gland and plays an important role in controlling water balance. Despite its name it probably has little to do with blood pressure control under normal circumstances. This is due to the fact that its vasoconstrictor actions are buffered by the baroreceptors that cause reflex changes in cardiac output so that there is little change in blood pressure.

Cortisol

Cortisol is secreted by the adrenal gland and appears to have a direct pressor effect on vascular tissues as well as an indirect effect through its slight mineralocorticoid action on the kidney. At the same time, high cortisol levels may cause a rise in circulating renin and, thereby, angiotensin II. Patients with excess cortisol secretion (Cushing's disease) have an increase in blood pressure. By contrast, when the adrenals fail, as occurs in Addison's disease, both cortisol and aldosterone levels are low and patients present with sodium and water depletion, low blood

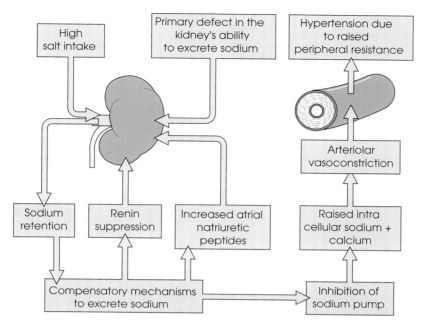

Figure 4.4
Suggested mechanism by which high salt intake causes high blood pressure.

pressure and postural falls in pressure, together with high plasma potassium and low plasma sodium levels.

Local vasoactive hormones

Prostaglandins

Prostaglandins are local tissue hormones that may play an important role in determining local arteriolar tone. When given by intravenous infusion, most prostaglandins cause vasodilatation. This is particularly so for prostacyclin. However, there is no evidence that there is any abnormality of prostaglandin metabolism in patients with high blood pressure. Despite this, indomethacin, an inhibitor of prostaglandin production, does block some of the effects of antihypertensive drugs, which suggests that some of these drugs may in part work through this local hormonal system.

Kallikrein–kinin system

The kallikrein–kinin system is a cascade system that produces bradykinin, a local tissue vasodilator, that could possibly lower blood pressure. Bradykinin is partly degraded by the same converting enzyme (ACE) that is responsible for the generation of angiotensin II. Thus ACE inhibitors could work both by reducing plasma angiotensin

II production and by increasing bradykinin levels, although it is probable that the fall in plasma angiotensin II is the main mode of action.

Nitric oxide (EDRF)

The powerful local vasodilator, nitric oxide, is secreted by endothelial cells lining the arterioles. Studies with inhibitors of the system have shown that it plays an important role in maintaining resting vascular tone, and some evidence suggests that in damaged arterioles, particularly in patients with atheroma, its release may be impaired, causing further vasoconstriction.

Endothelin

Endothelin is a peptide that is also secreted by endothelial cells and is the most powerful vasoconstrictor known. It has a long half-life and circulates at very low plasma levels. Its physiological role outside a local response to tissue injury is not at present clear.

Baroreceptor reflexes

The baroreceptors in the carotid sinus and aortic arch are sensitive buffers smoothing out variations in heart rate, blood pressure and cardiac output. In patients with high blood pressure there is some resetting of these baroreceptors, so that higher pressures are needed to activate the baroreceptor reflex, but there is no evidence that abnormal baroreceptor tone is responsible for high blood pressure. The abnormalities described to date are more likely to be a consequence of the chronically raised blood pressure, rather than the cause.

The kidney

Despite our knowledge of the various mechanisms that maintain normal blood pressure, studies of these systems have so far shed little light on the mechanism underlying essential hypertension. In the early 1960s it was suggested that in essential hypertension there might be a primary abnormality of the kidney, causing sodium and water retention. This would cause an increase in extracellular volume and a consequent rise in plasma volume and, therefore, a rise in cardiac output. The hypothesis suggested that this then caused an increase in peripheral resistance by autoregulation. Blood pressure then increased with a subsequent return of cardiac output to normal. The increase in blood pressure then caused further structural thickening of the small arterioles, giving rise to further vasoconstriction and the development of high blood pressure. This idea, whilst implicating the kidney as the main cause of hypertension, has not received much support as it has been difficult to demonstrate any evidence of plasma or extracellular volume expansion in the early phase of hypertension.

However, the concept that the kidney plays an important role in the development of hypertension has been illustrated by elegant kidney cross-transplantation experiments in rats with genetically determined hypertension. If the kidney from the genetically bred hypertensive rat is transplanted into a control animal, that animal then develops high blood pressure. If the reverse is done, and a kidney from a normotensive rat is put into a genetically hypertensive rat, that rat no longer develops high blood pressure. These experiments clearly demonstrate, at least in these rat models of hypertension, that the kidney is the primary cause of high blood pressure.

Much circumstantial evidence in humans also suggest that the kidney carries the basic underlying abnormality causing essential hypertension. For instance, human renal transplant recipients who receive a kidney from a donor with a family history of hypertension have been shown to have higher blood pressure than those receiving a kidney from a donor with a negative family history. Patients have also been described who developed renal failure secondary to essential hypertension who, when their own kidneys were removed and they received a successful renal transplant, developed normal blood pressure. These two findings support the concept that the kidney has a central role in the pathogenesis of essential hypertension in humans. Experiments in rats also suggest that the genetic abnormality in the kidney expresses itself as a difficulty in excreting sodium, and it is possible that this may underly essential hypertension in humans.

Other natriuretic hormones

This concept can be taken further. If the kidney is responsible for the development of high blood pressure, and the abnormality in the kidney is related to a difficulty in excreting sodium, then subjects who inherit this abnormality will, on a high-salt diet, tend to retain more sodium. This will stimulate greater compensatory mechanisms to get rid of the extra sodium and water. These compensatory mechanisms may include the atrial natriuretic peptides, which have been found to be raised in many patients with essential hypertension, and may involve other sodium excreting mechanisms, which could themselves, in the longer term, cause a rise in arteriolar tone and peripheral resistance.

One hypothesis is that a sodium transport inhibitor which slows down the sodium–potassium pump lining cell membranes, is increased in essential hypertension. This would give rise to an increase in intracellular sodium, which would increase intracellular calcium and thereby cause an increase in peripheral resistance.

Recently, a substance very similar to ouabain, a candidate for a sodium transport inhibitor has been isolated from human plasma, but whether this plays an important role in essential hypertension is not known. This hypothesis, therefore, requires further substantiation as there is considerable debate about the nature and actions of sodium transport inhibitors. Nevertheless, the overall concept does help to explain how a high salt intake can cause high blood pressure.

SECONDARY HYPERTENSION

The nature and investigation of underlying renal or adrenal diseases that are major causes of secondary hypertension are discussed in detail in Chapter 8.

Excess aldosterone (primary aldosteronism)

This is due to the autonomous oversecretion of the adrenal mineralocorticoid aldosterone, usually from a benign adrenal tumour (adenoma) or from bilateral enlargement of both adrenals. The excess aldosterone causes sodium retention and potassium loss. In this condition, plasma levels of renin and angiotensin II are low and plasma aldosterone levels are raised. After removal of the adrenal adenoma or blockade of aldosterone by the specific antagonist, spironolactone, blood pressure returns to normal or near normal in most patients.

Excess renin

Excess renin secretion can occur in renovascular and malignant hypertension. This is due to ischaemia, causing a reduction in perfusion pressure to the glomeruli, and the inappropriate secretion of excess renin and angiotensin II. Very rare tumours have also been described that secrete renin. These occur in the kidney and lead to very high circulating levels of renin and angiotensin II. If they are removed blood pressure returns to normal.

However, in some forms of renal disease and in patients with polycystic kidney disease, there may be subtle abnormalities of the renin–angiotensin system in relation to sodium balance. Plasma levels of angiotensin II may be inappropriately raised for the degree of sodium balance, and these two factors in combination could be responsible for high blood pressure.

Excess adrenaline or noradrenaline

Excess levels of these hormones are produced by phaeochromocytomas and other neuroendocrine tumours. Classically, the tumour causes intermittent release of noradrenaline and adrenaline, causing palpi-tations, headaches, sweating attacks, anxiety and very high blood pressures, which are directly due to the very high levels of these hormones.

FURTHER READING

Ching GWK, Beevers DG. Hypertension. *Postgrad Med J* 1991; **67**: 230–46.

De Wardener HE, MacGregor GA. The relation of a circulating sodium transport inhibitor (the natriuretic hormone?) to hypertension. *Medicine* 1983; **62**: 310–26.

Folkow B. Cardiovascular structural adaptation; its role in the initiation and maintenance of primary hypertension. *Clin Sci* 1978; **55**: 3s-22s.

Gordon RD. Mineralocorticoid hypertension. *Lancet* 1994; **344**: 240–3.

Harrap, SB. Hypertension: genes versus environment. *Lancet* 1994; **344**: 169–71.

Laragh JH. Vasoconstriction–volume analysis for understanding and treating hypertension: the use of renin and aldosterone profiles. *Am J Med* 1973; **55**: 261–74.

Moncada S, Palmer RMJ, Higgs EA. Nitric oxide: physiology, pathophysiology, and pharmacology. *Pharmacol Rev* 1991; **43**: 109–42.

Sagnella GA, MacGregor GA. Atrial natriuretic peptides. *Quart J Med* 1990; **77**: 1001–7.

DRUG-INDUCED HYPERTENSION

BACKGROUND

A large variety of drugs either cause hypertension or interfere with blood pressure control. In an ideal world, it would be best to avoid these agents. However, in many cases this is not possible due to important intercurrent diseases. Where suitable alternatives cannot be found, it may be necessary to initiate or increase antihypertensive therapy.

ORAL CONTRACEPTIVES

Almost all women who take combined oral contraceptives sustain a small rise in blood pressure, but this is usually within the normal range and is not considered of clinical importance (Fig 5.1). About 5% of women, particularly those who take the high-dose oestrogen pill, develop diastolic blood pressures above 90 mmHg. In most of these women, however, blood pressure was already in the upper range of normal before starting the pill. More severe hypertension and even malignant hypertension have been reported occasionally in some patients. Apart from the height of the blood pressure before starting the pill, there do not seem to be any obvious criteria that predict who will sustain a significant rise in blood pressure. In particular, hypertension in previous pregnancies and pre-eclampsia do not appear to be important risk factors. There does not seem to be any close relationship between the rise in pressure on the pill and the rise in weight.

The changes in blood pressure are associated with changes in the renin–angiotensin system, with a rise in levels of plasma renin substrate and in the amount of circulating angiotensin II. There is also some evidence

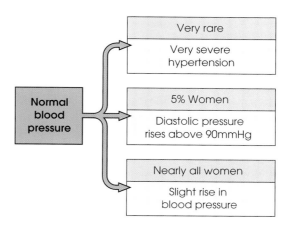

Figure 5.1

Changes in blood pressure in women taking oral contraceptive pills.

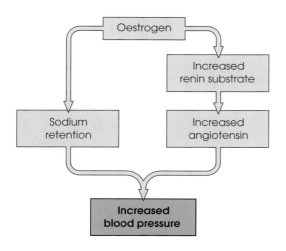

Figure 5.2
Mechanism of the rise in blood pressure
associated with oral contraceptive pill.

that there is volume expansion, and the combination of raised plasma angiotensin II and increased circulating volume may be the mechanism of the high blood pressure (Fig. 5.2). The lower dose oestrogen pill, more commonly used now, also raises blood pressure, although to a lesser extent. Some women who develop hypertension on the high-dose oestrogen pill may sustain a fall in pressure when the oestrogen content is reduced. There is increasing evidence that the progestogen-only contraceptive pill does not raise blood pressure and is probably preferable in those women who start with blood pressures in the upper range of normal, although this may be a less secure form of contraception.

If hypertension does develop on the pill, the patient should be advised to stop the combined pill and either change to a progestogen-only pill or alternative methods of birth control. However, there are some occasions when the cardiovascular or social risk from an unwanted pregnancy is so great that oral contraceptives have to be continued and antihypertensive drugs are given concurrently. All patients on the pill should have regular checks of their blood pressure at least once a year. The cardiovascular risk from the oral contraceptive is substantially worse in cigarette smokers, and in older women.

HORMONE REPLACEMENT THERAPY (HRT)

The effects of HRT on blood pressure were initially a cause for concern, but the majority of studies now indicate that there is no change in blood pressure (Fig. 5.3). The presence of mild to moderate hypertension is not a contraindication to HRT. Some evidence suggests that women on HRT have a lower overall cardiovascular risk profile than those not taking it. Women who are on treatment for high blood pressure or who have blood pressure in the upper normal range should not be denied the benefits of HRT. In a recent study of hypertensive women, HRT was discontinued, but after 3 months there was no change in their blood pressure. This strongly suggests that the HRT was not a factor in their blood pressure elevation in the first place. There is evidence that HRT leads to a reduction in coronary heart disease and overall mortality. The benefits of HRT, therefore, probably outweigh the risks in hypertensive women although unopposed oestrogens should not be used in women who have not had a hysterectomy owing to a small increase in the risk of endometrial cancer. Long-term HRT use may be associated with a small increase in the risk of breast cancer.

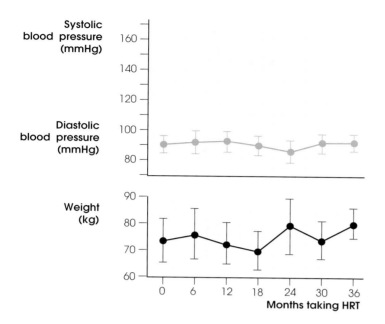

Figure 5.3
Sequential changes in blood pressure and weight in 75 hypertensive women starting hormone replacement therapy (HRT) (From Lip, Beevers, Churchill, 1994).

CARBENOXOLONE/LIQUORICE

Carbenoxolone is a liquorice-based drug that was used for the treatment of peptic ulcers. It blocks the action of the enzyme that protects mineralocorticoid receptors, thus allowing the normal levels of circulating cortisol to have a pronounced mineralocorticoid effect. This causes an identical syndrome to primary aldosteronism. The drug has now been replaced by the histamine antagonists (e.g. cimetidine etc.) and proton-pump inhibitors.

Liquorice has an identical action to carbenoxolone, and when eaten in excess can cause high blood pressure, hypokalaemia and oedema. Thiazide diuretics, when used to reduce the oedema, will cause further falls in plasma potassium and may cause muscle weakness and even paralysis. In some parts of Europe, particularly Holland, combined liquorice and salt tablets are eaten as sweets, which frequently cause high blood pressure. The combination of these sweets (Dubbel Zoote Drop) with the oral contraceptive is particularly dangerous.

ORAL AND TOPICAL CORTICOSTEROIDS

High-dose oral corticosteroid therapy raises blood pressure. This is, in part, due to the mineralocorticoid action of these high doses, causing sodium retention, but there is also an increase in plasma renin substrate and, thereby, increased levels of angiotensin II. Whether chronic low-dose steroid therapy with prednisolone in the treatment of rheumatoid arthritis or asthma causes an increase in blood pressure is more controversial. Nevertheless, all patients receiving prednisolone or other steroids need to have regular checks of their blood pressure as well as blood glucose and plasma electrolytes.

There are reports of hypertension developing with the use of high-dose topical steroid preparations for skin, ear and eye conditions. Some topical steroids have marked mineralocorticoid properties, causing sodium and water retention with hypokalaemia mimicking primary aldosteronism.

Several lines of evidence do suggest that steroids have an adverse effect on cardiovascular risk, not necessarily through high blood pressure, but probably as a result of a greater tendency to thrombosis. This needs to be borne in mind in patients on long-term steroids, particularly those who already have an adverse cardiovascular risk profile.

PURGATIVES AND DIURETICS

Purgatives do not cause hypertension but they may induce hypokalaemia, which may suggest the presence of either renal or adrenal disease. Unexplained hypokalaemia in a hypertensive patient can occasionally be due to purgative abuse and/or surreptitious vomiting. Diuretics remain the commonest cause of hypokalaemia, although this effect can be minimised if low doses are used. After stopping diuretics, serum potassium may take 1 month to return to normal.

If a patient develops profound hypokalaemia (e.g serum potassium below 3.0 mmol/l) whilst taking a low dose of a thiazide diuretic, then the clinician must investigate the possibility that there is another factor also lowering potassium levels. An underlying diagnosis of primary aldosterone excess should be considered. All patients with serum potassium levels of 3.5 mmol/l or below need detailed investigation.

COLD CURES

Many remedies for coughs and colds, and also some slimming pills, contain sympathomimetic amines that can raise blood pressure. The phenylamine group (ephedrine, pseudoephedrine, phenylephrine and phenylpropanolamine) all cause vasoconstriction, and hypertension has been reported in some patients. Hypertension may even be provoked or worsened by the overuse of nasal decongestant sprays. The imidazoline antifungal derivatives resemble clonidine in their chemical structure, and both hypertension and hypotension have been reported.

NEPHROTOXINS

Any drug that damages the kidney may cause a rise in blood pressure. For example, some antibiotics can cause renal failure, particularly the aminoglycosides (e.g. gentamicin) and some cephalosporins. This usually only occurs when they are given in high doses to patients who already have renal failure or are acutely ill. Phenacetin (an obsolete anti-inflammatory drug), when taken chronically, can cause renal papillary necrosis and eventually renal impairment. Because the damage is mainly in the medulla of the kidney, there is usually sodium loss. In general, patients with phenacetin nephropathy therefore had low rather than high blood pressure.

CYCLOSPORIN

Cyclosporin is a potent immunosuppressant used in patients with heart or kidney transplants, either in conjunction with steroids or other immunosuppressants, or on its own. However, it can cause both hepatic and renal impairment, although mild renal impairment often has to be accepted as a price to be paid for the better immunosuppression. The dose of the drug, therefore, has to be very carefully monitored.

Almost invariably, cyclosporin also causes a rise in blood pressure. This is, in part, related to renal impairment, but also seems to be related to sodium and water retention. Blood pressure in all patients needs to be carefully monitored and appropriate treatment given if the blood pressure does rise. It is claimed that calcium antagonists may be particularly effective in lowering blood pressure in cyclosporin-induced hypertension, but these drugs may also cause an increase in plasma cyclosporin levels.

ERYTHROPOETIN

Used in the treatment of the anaemia of chronic renal failure, erythropoetin leads to a significant rise in blood pressure in 30–35% of patients. The mechanisms of this pressor response are uncertain but may be related to a rise in haematocrit and increased total blood viscosity. In addition, erythropoetin may alter renal blood flow and stimu-

late renin release. Patients with chronic renal failure should not be denied the benefits of erythropoetin, but careful monitoring of blood pressure is mandatory, together where necessary with an increase in antihypertensive medication (see Chapter 14).

METHYSERGIDE

Fibrosis of the retroperitoneal tissues can occur with methysergide therapy for migraine. The ureters become obstructed and bilateral hydronephrosis and renal failure develop. The early beta-blocker practolol may also have caused retroperitoneal fibrosis, but there is no evidence that this is a problem with any beta-blocker available today.

MONOAMINE OXIDASE INHIBITORS (MAOI)

These powerful antidepressant drugs are not now widely used, but all of them may cause a sudden and occasionally disastrous rise in blood pressure if amines such as tyramine in cheese and yeast extracts are eaten, or decongestant 'cold cures' are taken.

TRICYCLIC ANTIDEPRESSANTS

These do not cause hypertension, but do interfere with the antihypertensive effects of the obsolete adrenergic neurone-blocking drugs, bethanidine and guanethidine. They may also cause serious arrhythmias, and their use in hypertensive patients should be discouraged, particularly if they have evidence of ischaemic heart disease.

LITHIUM

This agent is used on a long-term basis in manic or bipolar depression. The concurrent use of thiazide diuretics may increase the risk of lithium toxicity, so regular measurements of plasma lithium are necessary.

NON-STEROIDAL ANTI-INFLAMMATORY DRUGS (NSAIDS)

Indomethacin and all other NSAIDS relieve painful inflammation by blocking prostaglandin synthesis. They can also cause fluid retention and a rise in blood pressure. They block the antihypertensive action of thiazide diuretics as well as part of the action of the beta-blockers, some vasodilators and the ACE inhibitors, but they do not seem to affect the blood pressure-lowering capability of calcium antagonists. It has been claimed that the NSAID, sulindac, is the least likely to have adverse effects on blood pressure.

CLONIDINE WITHDRAWAL

Clonidine, a centrally acting alpha-stimulating drug, reduces blood pressure. However, when it is discontinued suddenly, a rebound rise in blood pressure occurs, which may be very severe and mimic a phaeochromocytoma crisis. Occasional rebound hypertension has also been reported with other centrally acting drugs, such as methyldopa. In our opinion, clonidine has no place in the treatment of hypertension and methyldopa should only be used for the treatment of hypertension in pregnancy.

TRACE METALS

Gold therapy can cause glomerulonephritis and hypertension. Both lead and cadmium as environmental pollutants have been implicated in causing hypertension. Recent evidence suggests that this is unlikely in the case with cadmium, but lead may be a cause of raised blood pressure. Both metals can cause renal damage when ingested in high doses in occupationally exposed workers.

DRUG ABUSE

During narcotic and alcohol withdrawal blood pressure rises to high levels. Marijuana will increase the heart rate but usually lowers the blood pressure. Cocaine can cause significant transient hypertension.

DRUG-INDUCED HYPOTENSION

Apart from the antihypertensive drugs discussed in Chapter 11, some other drugs may cause unwanted falls in blood pressure and some, particularly in overdosage, cause circulatory collapse. All tranquillisers and sedatives, particularly chlorpromazine derivatives and many opiate analgesics, may cause idiosyncratic or dose-related hypotension.

FURTHER READING

Dong W, Colhoun HM, Poulter NR. Blood pressure in women using oral contraceptives: results from the Heath Survey for England 1994. *J Hypertens* 1997; **15**: 1063–8.

Grossman E, Messerli FH. High blood pressure: a side effect of drugs, poisons and food. *Arch Intern Med* 1995; **155**: 450–60.

Lip GYH, Beevers M, Churchill D, *et al*. Hormone replacement therapy and blood pressure in hypertensive women. *J Hum Hypertens* 1994; **8**: 491–4.

Porter GA, Bennett WM, Sheps SG. Cyclosporin-associated hypertension. *Arch Intern Med* 1990; **150**: 280–3.

Raine AEG. Hypertension, blood viscosity, and cardiovascular morbidity in renal failure: implication for erythropoietin therapy. *Lancet* 1988; **1**: 97–9.

2

Section Two

6   BLOOD PRESSURE MEASUREMENT

BACKGROUND

The height of blood pressure is such an accurate predictor of an individual's future morbidity and mortality from cardiovascular disease that its measurement is the most important observation ever made in clinical practice. As blood pressure measurement is simple and carries no hazard, it should be regarded as a routine check to be carried out in everyone. Despite the importance of high blood pressure, there remains considerable confusion over the correct methods of measurement. Insufficient care is often taken with the technique, defective apparatus is often used and documentation is haphazard. However, the recent introduction of automatic and semi-automatic manometers, which do not employ a mercury column, has greatly improved the management of hypertensive patients.

HISTORY

The ancient Chinese Emperor Huang Ti (2000 b.c.) is credited with the first observation that people with full volume pulses develop strokes, and he also noted that people who eat a lot of salt have full volume pulses. He can, therefore, be regarded as the first person to appreciate the importance of estimating blood pressure, which he did by palpating the pulse and noting its character. In 1827, Richard Bright inferred that the blood pressure must be high when he observed that people dying of renal failure often had large hearts, but he had no blood pressure measurements to rely on.

The first recorded measurement of blood pressure was in 1733 by The Reverend Steven Hales, a distinguished biologist and the perpetual curate of Teddington, England. He introduced a cannula into an artery of a horse and measured the height of the column of blood rising up a glass tube. He observed that when the horse struggled, the blood pressure rose. This intra-arterial method of measuring blood pressure was perfected later by Sir George Pickering in humans, and has considerable research potential but no clinical value.

The indirect measurement of blood pressure was invented in 1896 by Scipione Riva Rocci. Using a mercury manometer, he was able to measure the pressure needed to occlude the brachial artery and obliterate the radial pulse. Riva Rocci's original apparatus subsequently underwent several modifications, but the basic principle remains the same to this day. The idea of listening below the occluded artery rather than just palpating it dates from 1905 when Nicolai Korotkov, a Russian army surgeon, wrote a thesis on the sounds that were audible as the mercury manometer was deflated. In honour of him, the blood pressure sounds are called the Korotkov sounds.

The oscillometric method of measuring blood pressure was introduced in 1890 by Michel Pachon. This technique relies on measuring the fluctuation in pressure within the air-filled cuff. The systolic and mean arterial pressures are thus measured accurately and the diastolic blood pressure is then calculated.

The advent of electronics has made possible the production of a great many automatic devices with varying degrees of accuracy. Some rely on the auditory technique of Korotkov and some on the oscillometric principles of Pachon. In normal practice, however, the mercury manometer remains the standard method and is attractive if only because of its simplicity and robustness. It is likely, however, that the use of mercury manometers will decline with improvements in electronic devices, and increasing concern about the environmental hazards of mercury.

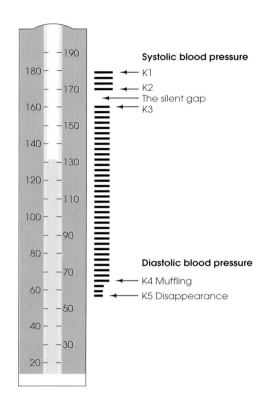

Figure 6.1
The Korotkov sounds.

THE KOROTKOV SOUNDS

After the cuff is inflated to the level that produces complete occlusion of the brachial artery, the column of mercury is allowed to fall at the rate of 2 mmHg/s. As the column falls, the various phases are heard through a stethoscope applied over the brachial artery. The exact physiological significance of the sounds is unclear, but their prognostic importance is undeniable. The Korotkov sounds are not transmitted heart sounds but are related to turbulence induced by constriction of the brachial artery (Fig. 6.1).

Phase 1. The first appearance of sounds. The systolic blood pressure is usually recorded when the second beat is heard on the grounds that the first beat might have been due to some form of extraneous noise.

Phase 2. The softening or disappearance of sounds.

The silent gap is usually no more than 5 mmHg and is frequently not present. When it is present it may lead to an underestimation of systolic blood pressure. It is thus very important to inflate the mercury column to 30 mmHg above that pressure needed to occlude the brachial pulse. The silent gap may be commoner in older patients with stiffer arteries.

Phase 3. The re-appearance of sounds.

These sounds are sometimes difficult to hear at first, but they become louder after 2 mmHg and assume a distinct tapping character.

Phase 4. Muffling of sounds.

The muffling of sounds used to be taken as the level of diastolic blood pressure. Often it is not easy to identify a distinct muffling phase, so phase 4 is no longer employed even in obstetric practice unless phase 5 cannot be identified.

Phase 5. The final disappearance of sounds.

Now regarded as the best measurement of diastolic blood pressure, the final disappearance of sounds is closer to the intra-arterial diastolic blood pressure.

In some patients with hyperdynamic circulations (for example in pregnancy, thyrotoxicosis, after exercise and in children), sounds may not completely disappear but may continue to be audible down to 0 mmHg. Sometimes this persistence of sounds is caused by tight clothing causing partial occlusion of the brachial artery above the cuff. More often than not, however, phase 4 and phase 5 diastolic blood pressures coincide, and a difference of more than 5 mmHg is unusual, even in pregnancy.

Brachial artery bruits

In some elderly patients, atheromatous narrowing of the brachial arteries means that there is a bruit over the artery, even when there is no compression applied by the cuff. Under these circumstances, it is necessary to record the phase 4 diastolic blood pressures. It is worth, however, measuring the blood pressure in the contralateral arm where there may be no bruit. Also in these circumstances, automatic oscillometric blood pressure measurement may be useful as this derives rather than measures the diastolic pressures.

UNITS OF BLOOD PRESSURE MEASUREMENT

The SI units of pressure measurement (kilopascals) have no place in the field of hypertension. If the SI units were to be introduced, the resultant confusion would endanger patient care.

Systolic or diastolic pressures

Most clinical research and randomised controlled trials have concentrated on the diastolic rather than the systolic blood pressure. There is really no good reason for this. Epidemiologists demonstrated 40–50 years ago that both systolic and diastolic blood pressure are potent predictors of risk. Furthermore, over the age of 45 years, the height of the systolic blood pressure predicts future morbidity and mortality more accurately than the diastolic blood pressure. Thus isolated systolic hypertension (ISH) is an important hazard to health, particularly in the elderly.

In 1991, the SHEP trial in the elderly demonstrated that the drug treatment of raised systolic blood pressure is of great clinical benefit even where the diastolic blood pressure is not raised. In 1997, this was confirmed in the multinational SYST–EUR trial (see Chapter 9).

It is likely, therefore, that over the next 10 years clinicians will increasingly concentrate their attention on the height of the systolic blood pressure. However, further research is necessary before confident recommendations on the value of systolic versus diastolic blood pressure reduction can be made in non-elderly patients.

Korotkov phase 4 or phase 5

Both diastolic phase 4 and phase 5 have been used for the estimation of diastolic blood pressure. Neither represents true diastolic blood pressure, which can only be measured by using an intra-arterial cannula. The indirect diastolic blood pressures are usually higher than the intra-arterial pressures, so it follows that phase 5 is closer to the true intra-arterial diastolic blood pressures. In clinical practice, diastolic blood pressures should normally be taken at phase 5, the disappearance of sounds. The reasons for this are:

- Most epidemiological studies of populations and cardiovascular risk have employed phase 5.
- All recent clinical trials on the treatment of hypertension have employed phase 5.
- Inter- and intra-observer variation is less when diastolic blood pressure is measured at phase 5.
- The assessment of when blood pressure sounds start to muffle is more subjective than when blood pressure sounds disappear completely.

Lying, sitting or standing

Normally, the diastolic blood pressure rises a little on standing, whilst the systolic blood pressure may fall by a few mmHg. Postural hypertension may occur in diabetics with autonomic neuropathy, and occasionally it is seen in elderly patients, particularly after meals. The obsolete adrenergic neurone-blocking drugs and the centrally acting alpha agonist, methyldopa, caused larger falls in standing as opposed to supine blood pressures.

It is probably wise, therefore, to measure blood pressure in the standing position at least once when assessing a new patient. If no postural drop is detected, lying or seated pressures can be employed thereafter. In diabetic patients, where there is a high risk of postural hypotension, blood pressure should routinely be measured in the standing and seated position.

All the large-scale epidemiological studies and almost all the randomised therapeutic controlled trials have employed seated diastolic blood pressure measurements. This is the most convenient position for routine clinical practice, and it is suggested, therefore, that lying blood pressures should not be measured as routine. The measurement of diastolic blood pressures with the subject seated has the added advantage that is then easier to ensure the cuff is at the same level as the heart.

Which arm?

Usually, there is no significant difference in pressures between the arms. Under these circumstances, it is best to use the nearest arm to the observer, as long as it is supported. Occasionally, especially in elderly people with extensive atheroma, there is a consistent difference between the two arms. If this is the case, blood pressure should routinely be measured in the arm with the highest pressure, with the appropriate documentation.

Mean arterial pressure

The mean arterial pressure can be calculated from the sum of the diastolic blood pressure plus one-third of the pulse pressure (systolic pressure minus diastolic pressure). It therefore takes into account both systolic and diastolic components of pressure. This calculated mean arterial pressure is closely related to the measured mean intra-arterial blood pressure. There is no reason to believe that mean arterial pressure has any greater physiological or pathological significance than either the systolic or diastolic blood pressures and for this reason it has little role in clinical practice.

Resting, casual or basal pressure

All blood pressures vary from minute to minute, day to day and season to season. There is a tendency for blood pressure variability to be greater in people with higher blood pressures, and systolic pressures vary more than diastolic. Data available from insurance companies and long-term observation surveys based on single casual blood-pressure measurements show that these measurements are very accurate predictors of future risk. When people relax in a quiet room, their blood pressures almost invariably fall, and even very high blood pressures associated with end-organ damage may settle considerably. Epidemiological studies have not been able to show that the basal blood pressure is of

any greater or lesser prognostic significance than the casual blood pressure, and the variability of blood pressure appears to have little significance at all.

However, recent studies employing 24-hour ambulatory blood pressure measurement (ABPM) tend to support the idea that blood pressures measured away from the clinical environment may be more predictive of risk than casual readings obtained during screening surveys or in clinical practice. No reliable long-term population surveys have yet tested out this relationship, but there is now fairly good evidence that blood pressures measured away from the clinical environment are more clearly related to left ventricular size as assessed by echocardiography.

White-coat hypertension

This term applies to patients whose blood pressure can be demonstrated to be raised only in the medical environment. If reliable evidence from 24-hour ABPM can unequivocally confirm that the blood pressure is completely normal at all stages except during a clinical consultation, then a diagnosis of white-coat hypertension is made. However, patients whose blood pressures are elevated in a clinical environment but normal while at home do require very careful observation and they cannot be regarded as 'normotensive'. Recent cross-sectional and follow-up studies strongly suggest that patients labelled as 'white-coat hypertensives' have left ventricular dimensions halfway between normotensive and mild hypertensive patients, and that the majority of such patients will develop sustained hypertension within 5 years. These patients, therefore, need careful, long-term follow-up.

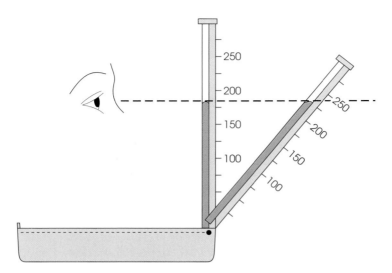

Figure 6.2
Blood pressure overestimation owing to faulty hinges.

All mild hypertensive patients should have their blood pressures measured at least twice on four consecutive occasions. Many patients' blood pressures settle if this is done. It is uncertain as to whether blood pressures measured frequently in the clinical environment as suggested above provide any more or less information than a 24-hour ABPM.

Blood pressure load

Recently, the concept of blood pressure load has been advanced. This implies that the number of raised blood pressure readings over a 24-hour period may be of prognostic significance. Thus, patients whose blood pressures settle at night ('dippers') have a lower 24-hour blood pressure load and may be at lower risk than patients classified as non-dippers.

BLOOD PRESSURE MEASUREMENT

Sources of error

Whilst blood pressure measurement is easy, it is also easy to make serious errors. These may lead to inappropriate diagnosis of hypertension or the inappropriate reassurance of patients who have genuinely raised blood pressures. We support the aphorism 'if you cannot measure something accurately, then measure it often'.

Errors due to the manometer

• Insufficient or too much mercury in the manometer so that at rest the mercury column does not read 0 mmHg.
• The mercury column slopes away from the vertical owing to damaged hinges on the manometer box (Fig. 6.2). This causes falsely elevated blood pressure

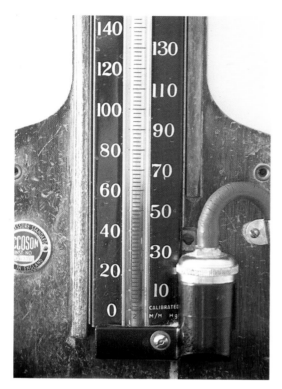

Figure 6.3
A dirty manometer tube (photographed when reading 0 mmHg) in a hospital casualty department.

readings. (Some manometers are manufactured with a built-in tilt and in these a correction is made with a slightly longer glass column.)

- The mercury column becomes dirty; as air is freely in contact with the mercury, mercuric oxide can form on the inside of the glass tubing so that the mercury meniscus can no longer be seen (Fig. 6.3). All glass tubing should be cleaned about once a year.
- If the rubber tubing is perished and leaky, this will cause over-rapid and

uncontrolled deflation of the cuff and may lead to falsely low blood pressure readings.

Errors caused by the cuff

Cuff size too small When the rubber bladder inside the cuff is too small, there is inadequate compression of the brachial artery. The cuff itself should be a minimum of 25 cm longer than the internal rubber bladder, with a tail of over 60 cm. Velcro cuffs have shorter tails and are convenient but they may tend to lose their grip unless they are cleaned regularly.

The rubber bladder inside the cuff should encircle about 80% of the arm circumference, and preferably more. Bladders that are too small cause over-reading of blood pressure. Unfortunately, most commercially available blood pressure cuffs have bladders that are too small.

The 'large adult' cuff does encircle a sufficient part of the circumference of the arm, but unfortunately its width (15 cm) means that it is often not possible to apply one's stethoscope over the brachial artery unless the patient has long arms as well as being obese.

In routine clinical practice, we now strongly recommend the 'alternative adult' cuff (Fig. 6.4). This has a rubber bladder that measures 12.5–13 cm × 33–35 cm. If this cuff is used in routine practice, it will only very rarely be necessary to employ a large adult cuff. The conventional adult cuff of 12.5 × 23 cm should now be phased out as it is unsuitable for measurement of blood pressure where the arm circumference exceeds 33 cm. A recent survey demonstrated that 7.5% of the general population and 15% of hypertensive patients have arm circumferences that exceed 33 cm, so the standard adult cuff would not provide accurate readings.

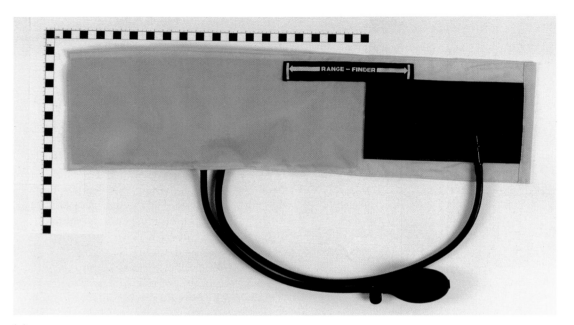

(a)

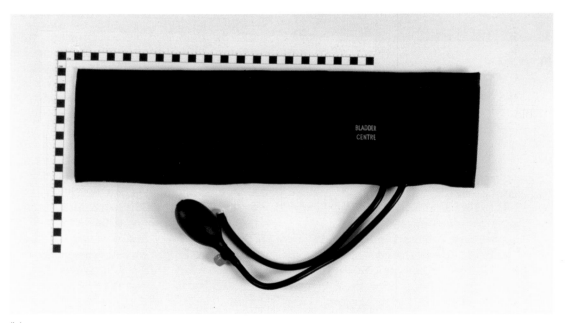

(b)

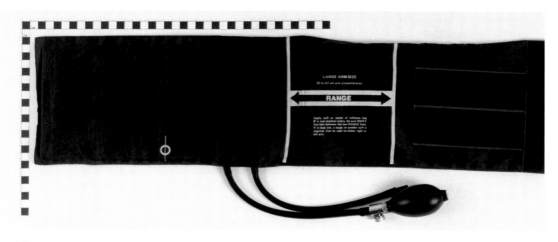

(c)

Figure 6.4
(a) The 'alternative adult' cuff with rubber bladder (13 x 35cm); now highly recommended for routine use.
(b) The 'normal adult' cuff with rubber bladder (13 x 23cm); only suitable if arm circumference is less than 33cm. (c) The 'large arm size' cuff with rubber bladder (15 x 30cm); useful if arm cirmcumference exceeds 33cm; however, it tends to extend into antecubital fossa unless the patient has long arms.

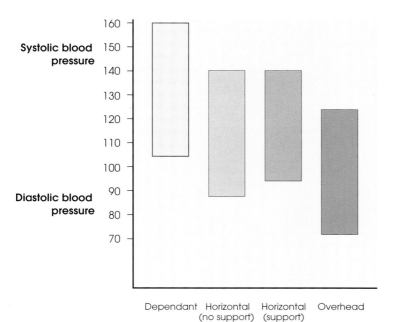

Figure 6.5
Effect of arm position on blood pressure.

The alternative adult cuff is now available through most manufacturers and is recommended for routine practice by the British Hypertension Society, and is also routinely used in Sweden.

There is some bacteriological hazard from the continued use of dirty blood pressure cuffs in hospital wards.

The cuff is not at the same level as the heart Whilst it does not matter where the mercury manometer is in relation to the heart (it should be as near as possible to the observer's eye), it is very important that the cuff is at the same level as the heart. If the arm is raised, falsely low readings are obtained and if the cuff is below heart level, falsely high readings are obtained (Fig. 6.5). It is also very important that the arm is supported, as the isometric exercise of holding the arm up can cause a rise in blood pressure. It is difficult to ensure the cuff is at the correct level when measuring lying or standing pressures.

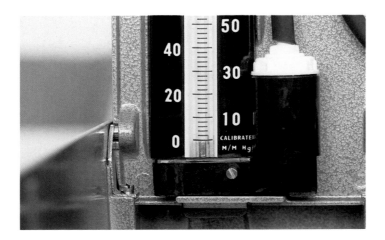

Figure 6.6

The correct technique for measuring blood pressure. (i) Ensure the mercury meniscus reads zero before use. The observer's eye must be level with the top of the meniscus to avoid parallax error.

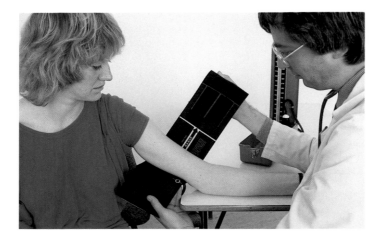

(ii) The φ mark must be over the brachial artery.

Faulty or blocked inflation/deflation devices If the inflation/deflation device is faulty, it is difficult to control the column of mercury as it falls, and this may lead to overestimation of blood pressure.

Observer errors

Faulty technique If the blood pressure cuff is not inflated high enough to occlude the brachial artery, systolic blood pressure is seriously underestimated. The clinician may falsely conclude that phase 3, the reappearance of systolic sounds, is the systolic blood pressure rather than phase 1.

Parallax error If the mercury column is not level with the observer's eye, a parallax error of up to 2 mmHg may occur.

Terminal digit preference This occurs when the observer reads either up or down to the nearest 5 or 10 mmHg. As the

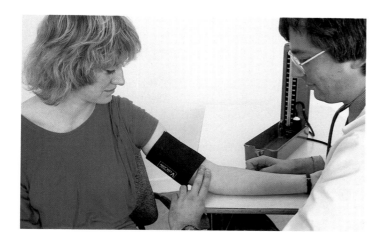

(iii) Ensure that there is enough space below the cuff so that the stethoscope does not come into contact with the cuff.

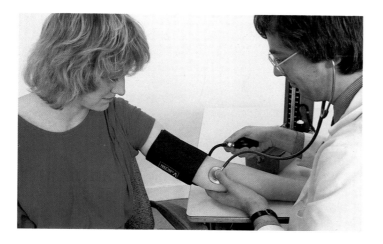

(iv) Use a stethoscope diaphragm to listen over the brachial artery.

markings on the glass tubings are in 2 mm intervals, it is not logical to measure blood pressure to the nearest odd number. This problem may not appear to matter too much in individual cases with severe hypertension, but it is very important when assessing mild hypertensive patients. It is also important in randomised controlled trials or population surveys. Systematic differences may be obtained between observers if one observer has a tendency to read up to the nearest 10 mmHg whilst the other has a tendency to read down to the nearest 10 mmHg. In view of the enormous importance of blood pressure in predicting individual survival, a very accurate blood pressure reading should be obtained. The blood pressure should, therefore, be measured to the nearest 2 mmHg.

Observer bias

If the observer is aware that the patient is receiving treatment, he may tend to bias readings to be lower to fulfill his preconceived notions. Observer bias must be abolished or minimised in randomised controlled trials and population surveys.

Hearing impairment

Hearing impairment will cause the observer to underestimate the systolic blood pressure and overestimate the diastolic blood pressure.

Male and female connectors

To avoid confusion and total interchangeability of cuffs and manometers, it is conventional for the manometer to have the male connection and the cuff to have the female connection. It is sensible for the clinician to have some spare connectors readily available.

CORRECT TECHNIQUE FOR MEASURING BLOOD PRESSURE (FIG. 6.6)

(1) Ensure the patient is seated comfortably leaning on the back of the chair and is neither too hot nor too cold. Blood pressures are lower in a warmer environment, and rise when it is cold. Try to avoid exertion and stressful discussions immediately before pressures are measured. If this is the patient's first ever test, it is wise to explain that there will be some slight discomfort as the cuff is inflated. Try to position the manometer so the patient is unable to see the mercury column.

(2) Apply the forearm cuff neatly, with the zero mark over the brachial pulse. Many modern cuffs have the 33 cm circumference marked out. If the arm circumference exceeds this range, a larger cuff should be used.

(3) Ensure that the manometer column is vertical and connect it to the cuff.

(4) Ensure the forearm is supported, preferably resting on a desk, slightly extended and externally rotated.

(5) Inflate the cuff at a slow steady rate to 30 mmHg above the level needed to occlude the radial or brachial pulse.

(6) Place the diaphragm of the stethoscope over the brachial artery. Do not press too hard. It does not matter if the diaphragm is partly underneath the edge of the cuff, although this can cause creaking noises that may confuse the observer.

(7) The observer's eyes should be at the same level as the top of the column of mercury.

(8) Deflate the manometer cuff at the rate of 2 to 3 mmHg/s.

(9) Record the systolic blood pressure (phase 1) when the blood pressure sounds are first heard.

(10) Record the diastolic pressure at phase 5 (disappearance of sounds). If sounds can still be heard, even when the manometer reads 30 mmHg or less, then diastolic pressures should be taken at the muffling of sounds (phase 4).

(11) Blood pressures should be measured to the nearest 2 mmHg.

(12) Write down all the readings immediately.

(13) At first consultation check the blood pressure in both arms to ensure there is no discrepancy. If pressures differ significantly there may be atheromatous narrowing of the subclavian artery causing falsely low pressure readings. In this case the arm with the higher pressure should be used thereafter.

(14) Measure the blood pressure at least twice at all consultations. The second reading is the one on which decisions are usually made.

Special situations

Atrial fibrillation

Atrial fibrillation renders blood pressure difficult to measure accurately. At least three readings should be taken on each occasion.

Pregnancy

It has been argued that when measuring blood pressure in pregnant women, it is 'common' to be unable to identify the fifth phase as, due to hyperdynamic circulation of pregnancy, sounds are audible over the brachial artery even when there is no arm compression. However, a recent comparison of pregnant versus non-pregnant women has shown that there is little difference in the gap between muffling and disappearance of diastolic sounds in pregnancy. This and other observations mean that diastolic blood pressures in pregnancy should also be measured at the fifth phase and not at the fourth phase. A recent survey demonstrated considerable confusion amongst obstetricians, half of whom employed phase 4 and half phase 5.

It should be remembered that in obstetrical practice, automatic blood pressure machines are often employed and these, whether oscillometric or auditory, all measure diastolic blood pressure at the fifth phase. It is reasonable, therefore, for clinicians to adopt the same technique as the equipment they employ.

Aortic coarctation

There is evidence that aortic coarctation is underdiagnosed. Where the foot pulses are unobtainable, weak or delayed, routine measurement of blood pressure in the legs is strongly advocated. This is a simple technique. The patient, where relevant, must remove trousers and lie prone. An appropriate thigh cuff is applied and the stethoscope placed in the popliteal fossa. Readings are then taken in the same way as in the arms.

Children

The measurement of blood pressure should be an integral part of the assessment of a paediatric patient. The principles are no different from those used in adults. In children over the age of three, a conventional mercury manometer is used and the Korotkov sounds auscultated. If the Korotkov sounds prove inaudible, the systolic pressure can be measured by palpation alone. In infants, in whom conventional measurements are impossible, Doppler blood pressure measuring devices should be used.

MEASURING DEVICES

Anaeroid sphygmomanometers

Anaeroid sphygmomanometers are useful, and when new are usually accurate, although it is sometimes difficult to obtain a reliable reading when the needle flickers. They tend to deteriorate after 2 or 3 years, however, and there is no way of telling whether they are accurate except by checking them against a mercury manometer with a Y-tube connection to a cuff wrapped around a bottle.

It is, therefore, best not to use anaeroid sphygmomanometers in hospitals, clinics or health centres, where the mercury manometer is preferable. Anaeroid manometers are, however, more portable and so are useful for home visits.

The random-zero sphygmomanometer

The Hawksley random-zero sphygmomanometer is based on the same principle as the conventional manometer but is designed to minimise at least some systematic error and abolish observer bias. This equipment has been used in many population surveys and randomised controlled trials of drug therapy. The system relies on a mercury reservoir of variable size, so the clinician is unaware of the level of mercury that is zero when measuring the pressure. After the manometer is disconnected from the cuff, the column mercury falls to a figure that is meant to be randomly distributed between 0 and 60 mmHg (0–20 mmHg in the USA). Recent evidence has suggested that the random zero is not randomly distributed although it remains unpredictable.

London School of Hygiene Sphygmomanometer

Heavy and expensive, but reliable, the London School of Hygiene Sphygmomanometer is powered by cylinders of carbon dioxide. It did provide accurate measures of blood pressure in a totally unbiased manner, but it is now hardly used.

Automated manometers

A great many automatic electronic blood pressure measuring devices are now available. In general, the clinician armed with a well-maintained conventional mercury manometer has no need for other more expensive equipment. Many electronic devices are marketed but, with some exceptions, most are inaccurate. Unless there are published data available on a particular apparatus, demonstrating that readings are closely matched to those of a mercury manometer, the clinician should avoid these types of equipment.

Automatic machines, such as the OMRON HEM 705CP, that print and date the measurement are very useful as they allow the patient to keep an accurate record of their blood pressure over a period of time.

The OMRON device has passed tests of accuracy suggested by the British Hypertension Society.

Unfortunately, some automated blood pressure systems are marketed where no attempt has been made to produce any form of standardisation or accuracy testing. If patients are keen to measure their blood pressures at home, they should be encouraged to use validated machines. If other automated devices are used, patients should be advised to bring them to the clinic for checking.

Automatic manometers can be employed to measure blood pressure repeatedly at intervals of between 30 seconds and one hour. These instruments are expensive but, if they are reliable, they are useful during infusion studies and after test doses of drugs, such as the ACE inhibitors, in patients with severe hypertension or heart failure. Similarly, they are useful as an alternative to 24-hour ABPM. A patient who may have 'white-coat hypertension' may benefit from being left in a quiet room with an automatic machine, and having their blood pressure measured every half an hour for 2–3 hours. Very often, the blood pressure will settle as the patient relaxes away from the formal clinical environment.

As stated earlier, advances in technology will lead to the availability of an increasing number of reliable semi-automatic devices and possibly, in time, the mercury manometer will be rendered obsolete.

INTRA-ARTERIAL BLOOD PRESSURE

This invasive technique for measuring blood pressure is mainly used in research units, and cannot be applied generally. All the prognostic and therapeutic information available on high blood pressure and its treatment is based on the indirect cuff method, and the prognostic significance of the lower ambulatory intra-arterial pressure is uncertain. The technique is also not without hazard.

NON-INVASIVE AMBULATORY BLOOD PRESSURE MEASUREMENTS (ABPM)

There is increasing interest in the assessment of blood pressure away from the stressful environment of the clinic or hospital. In general, home blood pressures are lower than clinic readings. Many ambulatory automated non-invasive manometers are now coming into use. However, the fact remains that accurate but 'casual' pressure readings obtained by a doctor are a very reliable guide to prognosis, and the meaning of lower readings obtained at other times is uncertain.

The 24-hour ambulatory technique has, however, drawn attention to so-called 'white-coat hypertension'. The main problem is that there has as yet been no formal epidemiological assessment of the prognostic significance of ambulatory blood pressure measurement (ABPM) compared with accurate 'clinical' recordings. One long-term, follow-up study suggests that ambulatory blood pressure readings predict survival better than conventional clinical (office) blood pressure measurements, although the measurement techniques used in that study are no longer generally available.

The main problem faced by the clinician is that patients whose pressures are persistently elevated in the clinical environment cannot be regarded as being without risk simply because their pressures are 'normal' when at home. However, ABPM does have a role in assessing some mild hypertensive patients who have absolutely no evidence of end-organ damage and who appear agitated or distressed, particularly at hospital attendance.

Whatever happens, however, patients with 'white-coat hypertension' need careful long-term follow-up even though they may not immediately require antihypertensive drug therapy. ABPM, with its large number of reliable measurements, can sometimes be used to 'prove' to reluctant or doubting patients that they really do have sustained hypertension requiring treatment.

The Spacelabs 90207 automatic blood pressure system has passed tests for accuracy and is now commonly used.

TRAINING OF OBSERVERS

Both medical and nursing students are taught blood pressure measurement at an early stage of their careers. However, they are often taught by non-clinicians in physiology classes and there is no re-training thereafter. Many surveys have shown that there is a disastrous state of confusion about the correct method of measuring blood pressure and the assessment of the diastolic pressure (muffling versus disappearance of sounds).

It is essential, therefore, that all junior doctors and trained nursing staff should be re-trained in blood pressure measurement using the methods described here. When major national or international surveys or trials are contemplated, again the re-training and certification of observers is mandatory if systematic errors or biases are to be avoided.

Several video-cassette recordings are now available, which emphasise the correct techniques and display a series of falling columns of mercury, together with the Korotkov sounds. They are highly recommended, and should be standard equipment in every school of medicine or nursing, as well as in primary health care teams and specialist blood pressure groups.

FURTHER READING

British Hypertension Society. British Hypertension Society recommendations on blood pressure measurement. *Br Med J* 1986; **293**: 611.

Churchill D, Beevers DG. Has the random zero sphygmomanometer been exonerated? *J Hum Hypertens* 1997; **11**: 73–4.

Joint National Committee on Detection, Evaluation, and Treatment of High Blood Pressure. The Sixth Report of the Joint National Committee on Prevention, Detection, Evaluation and Treatment of High Blood Pressure (JNC VI). *Arch Intern Med* 1997; **157**: 2413–46.

O'Brien E. A century of confusion; which bladder for accurate blood pressure measurement? *J Hum Hypertens* 1996; **10**: 565–72.

O'Brien E, O'Malley K. Blood pressure measurement. In Birkenhäger WH and Reid JL, eds, *Handbook of Hypertension*, vol 14. Amsterdam: Elsevier, 1991.

Pickering TG, Harshfield GA, Devereux RB, *et al.* What is the role of ambulatory blood pressure monitoring in the management of hypertensive patients? *Hypertension* 1985; **7**: 171–7.

THE ASSESSMENT OF A NEW PATIENT

BACKGROUND

Usually, new hypertensive patients are detected during the course of a routine medical examination for employment or insurance or during some sort of case detection programme or screening survey. Many are diagnosed during a consultation for an unrelated condition. Unfortunately, a significant number of patients remain undiagnosed until a late stage of their disease for example when they sustain a heart attack or a stroke. This should not happen, as early detection and management can prevent many of these vascular complications. In women, hypertension may be detected by obstetricians during pregnancy or while following up patients receiving the oral contraceptive. It is logical, however, to check the pressure of all patients seeking any form of medical aid as this simple measurement has such important preventive implications. All subjects who either have a diastolic pressure greater than 90 mmHg or a systolic pressure greater than 160 mmHg should then undergo further assessment.

CLINICAL HISTORY

In the absence of vascular complications most patients are usually symptomless. Symptoms due to raised blood pressure itself are rare, but there remains a common misconception among patients and relatives that high blood pressure makes them feel unwell. In the majority it is simply a risk factor for premature cardiovascular disease, which has been labelled the 'silent killer' because of its early asymptomatic course. Once diagnosed, patients may then become unwell due to the anxiety induced by the act of diagnosis.

All patients should be asked whether they have ever had their blood pressure measured before and if they can remember the level. In particular, women should be questioned about their blood pressure in pregnancy.

Headache

Headaches do sometimes occur in very severe hypertension and in patients with malignant phase hypertension due to raised intracranial pressure. Otherwise, migraine and tension headaches, whilst troublesome, are not related to the high blood pressure.

Breathlessness

Left ventricular failure with orthopnoea and paroxysmal nocturnal dyspnoea may be due to hypertension alone, particularly in the accelerated or malignant phase. It may also be related to concomitant coronary heart disease. Asthma and chronic obstructive airways disease are common, but not associated with hypertension. When present, these diagnoses are important as they influence the choice of antihypertensive drugs. Patients with asthma should not receive beta-blockers, so ACE inhibitors, angiotensin-receptor blockers, calcium-channel blockers or thiazide diuretics should be used instead (see Chapter 14).

Chest pain

Chest pain may be due to angina or a heart attack, both of which are complications of hypertension.

Palpitations

A history of recurrent episodes of tachycardia raises the possibility of phaeochromocytoma, although it may also be due to intrinsic cardiac disease, anxiety or thyrotoxicosis. Alcohol excess can cause arrhythmias and raised blood pressure.

Intermittent claudication

Aortic or femoral atheroma are complications of hypertension and, when present, beta-blockers are contraindicated. Furthermore, patients with arterial disease may also have atheromatous renal artery stenosis, particularly if they are cigarette smokers.

Polyuria and nocturia

Polyuria and nocturia can occur with intrinsic renal disease, which may cause hypertension or may follow renal damage secondary to the raised blood pressure. Nocturia also occurs in men with advancing age due to prostatic hypertrophy. The calcium-channel blockers themselves, particularly the dihydropyridines such as nifedipine and amlodipine, can cause nocturia, and it is important not to confuse this with prostatic hypertrophy. Alpha-blockers can cause or aggravate stress incontinence in women.

Diabetes mellitus

Patients with diabetes are more prone to hypertension and its vascular complications. The presence of diabetes substantially influences the management of hypertension (see Chapter 14); in particular, diuretics should be avoided in diabetic patients as they may cause or aggravate glucose intolerance, and ACE inhibitors or angiotensin-receptor blockers are the preferred option.

Visual symptoms

Visual loss may occur in hypertension if there are retinal haemorrhages or exudates due to accelerated or malignant hypertension. Central or branch retinal vein thrombosis and retinal artery occlusion are strongly associated with hypertension, as well as cigarette smoking. Amaurosis fugax may result from embolus formation from carotid artery stenosis. There may also be visual disturbance due to transient cerebral ischaemia or strokes.

Neurological symptoms

Transient or persistent hemiplegia may be due to cerebral haemorrhage or infarction, both of which are complications of hypertension. Hypertensive patients are at risk of subarachnoid haemorrhage, particularly if they have polycystic kidney disease or are smokers.

PAST HISTORY

It is important to take an accurate past history, particularly seeking for renal disease or evidence of previous vascular complications of raised blood pressure. In women, a detailed obstetric history is necessary. Previous pre-eclampsia or pregnancy-induced hypertension, or raised pressure whilst receiving the oral contraceptive, are important. There is an association between pregnancy-induced hypertension and raised blood pressure in later life.

FAMILY HISTORY

Frequently, patients do not know whether their parents or siblings had hypertension,

but useful indicators in the family history are premature death from heart attack or stroke. Essential hypertension does run in families, as does polycystic kidney disease, which is inherited as a autosomal dominant condition. This particularly should be considered where there is a strong family history of hypertension, subarachnoid haemorrhage or renal failure.

Diabetes mellitus

Diabetes, particularly maturity onset diabetes, does appear to be partly familial, and is strongly associated with hypertension.

Relatives of hypertensive patients

Patients should always be advised to tell their relatives to have their blood pressures checked.

SOCIAL HISTORY

The epidemiology of hypertension is discussed in Chapter 3. Some aspects are especially relevant to the individual case.

Occupation

Hypertension is more common in people in the lower socio-economic groups, but is not associated with any particular occupational groups and is not necessarily associated with stressful jobs. The social class link may be explained by the higher prevalence of obesity and a higher intake of alcohol and salt and in people in lower socio-economic groups. Some hypertensive patients show a very marked pressor response to stress at home or at work and detailed questioning may reveal this. The evidence that psychosocial stress causes chronic elevation of blood pressure is poor and reliable studies have demonstrated no association.

High alcohol intake

Heavy drinking is closely related to high blood pressure, independent of age, sex, personality, cigarette smoking, obesity or salt consumption. Alcoholics and heavy drinkers are frequently hypertensive and their blood pressure settles without drugs if they stop drinking. Detailed questioning on drinking habits is necessary in all hypertensive patients. It is best to document the total number of units of alcohol consumed in an average week.

Salt intake

Patients should be asked whether they consume much salt and particularly if they add it at table or in cooking. Many processed foods have a high salt content and patients who eat out or consume fast foods are likely to have quite high salt intakes. However, many patients underestimate their salt intake, which can be shown by 24-hour measurement of sodium excretion.

Fat intake

The amount of saturated animal and vegetable fat in the diet is an important determinant of serum cholesterol levels, which are one of the three major risk factors for premature cardiovascular disease. It is important therefore to question all patients about the amount of fat in their diet.

Calorie intake

Many patients with high blood pressure are overweight and it is important to try to get some idea of their calorie intake in order to advise them how best to lose weight.

Cigarette smoking

An independent cardiovascular risk factor, cigarette smoking is not related to high blood pressure, but when these two independent risk factors are present together, the degree of risk is compounded. Patients who smoke are more likely to develop peripheral vascular disease, renal artery stenosis and malignant hypertension.

DRUG HISTORY

Antihypertensive drugs

Often hypertensive patients are receiving unnecessarily complicated drug combinations. Many patients do not know what their tablets are or what they are for. At a clinical assessment where the previous drug history is not known, patients should be asked to bring all their tablets with them. There is often an alarming difference between the treatment the doctor thinks the patient is receiving and the tablets the patient actually takes. Patients should be given special cards or booklets that list drug names and doses as well as blood pressure measurements. These can be written in by any doctor or nurse who manages the patient, and this greatly improves liaison between the family and hospital doctors. (See Chapter 13).

Other medications

Some drugs, notably oral contraceptives and carbenoxolone, can cause hypertension. Some psychotropic drugs and NSAIDs inter-react with antihypertensive drugs (see Chapters 5 and 11).

EXAMINATION

Breathlessness, distress and anxiety may be present in hypertensive patients who are unwell. The following features suggest specific diagnoses relevant to raised blood pressure:

Patient appearance

Plethoric facies

A plethoric appearance suggests polycy-thaemia, which is itself associated with raised blood pressure. It also occurs in patients with excessive alcohol intake, heavy cigarette smoking and Cushing's syndrome.

Cushingoid appearance

Cushing's syndrome may cause hypertension (see Chapter 8) as does corticosteroid therapy. Occasionally, the alcoholic pseudo-

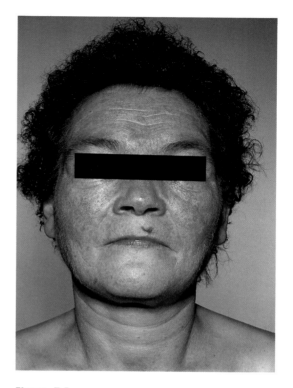

Figure 7.1
Patient with alcoholic pseudo–Cushing's syndrome.

Cushing's syndrome is present and other stigmata of liver disease should be looked for (Fig. 7.1).

Sweating, tremor, restlessness and anxiety

These symptoms raise the possibility of hyperthyroidism, which may cause raised systolic blood pressure. Phaeochromo-cytoma or simple anxiety itself can also cause these symptoms. Some patients become very stressed when they visit their doctor or attend hospital clinics and they exhibit some of these symptoms and have falsely raised blood pressure.

Blanching and pallor

Together with weight loss, sweating and tachycardia, blanching and pallor raise the possibility of phaeochromocytoma. Most patients with this condition have persistently raised blood pressure but there may be marked fluctuations and even episodes of hypotension.

Obesity

Obesity is associated with raised blood pressure, which is compounded by a tendency to overestimate the blood pressure in obese arms when an inappropriately small cuff is used (see Chapter 6). Body weight should be checked as well as height. In obese patients it is useful to plot weight in relation to height or to calculate the Body Mass Index (BMI), which is the weight in kilograms divided by the height in metres squared.

BMI > 30 Kg/m²	obese
BMI 25–29 Kg/m²	overweight
BMI < 25 Kg/m²	acceptable
BMI < 20 Kg/m²	underweight

However, BMI does not take into account the distribution of body fat. Central obesity in men may be a more powerful predictor of cardiovascular risk and is frequently associated with glucose intolerance. Some clinicians routinely measure waist/hip ratio to diagnose central obesity.

Acromegaly

About 50% of patients with acromegaly are hypertensive (Fig. 7.2).

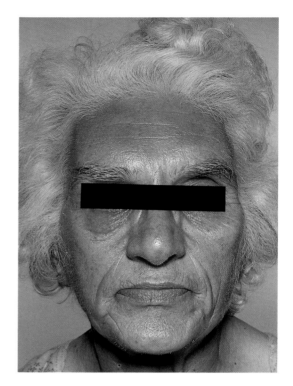

Figure 7.2
Patient with acromegaly and hypertension.

Neurofibromatosis (von Recklinghausen's disease)

Multiple neurofibromata and cafe au lait spots suggest neurofibromatosis, which is associated with both phaeochromocytoma and renal artery stenosis (Fig. 7.3).

The cardiovascular system

Blood pressure

The correct technique for measuring blood pressure is covered in Chapter 6. Pressures

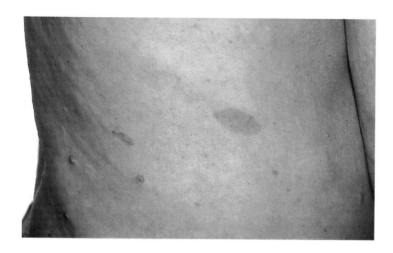

Figure 7.3
Patient with von Recklinghausen's neurofibromatosis.

should be measured at least once in both arms. Seated blood pressures are best employed when assessing patients but pressures should also be measured standing if the patient, is diabetic or complains of postural dizziness. This may particularly occur in the elderly, in patients with phaeochromocytoma, and in those receiving the outdated adrenergic-blocking drugs.

Atrial fibrillation renders blood pressure measurement difficult due to the fact that blood pressure will vary from beat to beat. Several readings should be taken. It may be due to hypertension alone or caused by coronary heart disease, alcoholic cardiomyopathy, thyroid disease or rheumatic heart disease.

blockers or it may be due to myxoedema or to heart block. An ECG should be obtained before any drugs are given (beta-blockers and verapamil may make heart block worse). All peripheral pulses should be checked and the carotid and femoral pulses auscultated for bruits. The femoral pulse should always be checked once against the brachial or radial pulse to detect radial–femoral delay or a disparity in volume, suggesting coarctation of the aorta or severe aortic atheroma.

Osler's manoeuvre to assess arterial wall thickness when the cuff is inflated above systolic blood pressure has now been shown to be unhelpful.

The pulse

Classically in hypertension the pulse has a large volume, but this is not a reliable sign. Tachycardia suggests anxiety, thyrotoxicosis or, very rarely, phaeochromocytoma. Bradycardia is most commonly due to beta-

Cardiac apex

The position of the cardiac apex should be measured and the presence of a left ventricular heave noted. The presence of left ventricular hypertrophy (LVH) is a potent predictor of risk in hypertensive patients.

Heart sounds

In patients with raised blood pressure, the aortic component of the second heart sound is loud. If there is clinical or subclinical left ventricular failure, a third sound or even a combined third and fourth sound (gallop rhythm) may be heard.

Cardiac murmurs are assessed in the conventional manner; hypertension can exist with mitral valve disease and with aortic stenosis with or without regurgitation.

Aortic systolic murmurs of no haemodynamic significance are common in hypertension. If, however, the aortic component of the second heart sound is quiet, aortic stenosis should be considered, particularly if there is evidence of disproportionate LVH. Aortic systolic murmurs associated with a loud second heart sound are likely to be due to aortic sclerosis, which is particularly common in the elderly.

Coarctation of the aorta is usually associated with loud systolic murmurs over most of the left precordium into the left scapular region.

The respiratory system

The presence of basal pulmonary crepitations suggestive of left ventricular failure, or of rhonchi suggesting obstructive airways disease, strongly influences the choice of antihypertensive drugs. With airway obstruction, beta-blockers are absolutely contraindicated (see Chapter 11).

The abdomen

The presence of hepatomegaly raises the possibility of liver disease caused by alcohol abuse, although in decompensated cirrhosis with jaundice or ascites, hypertension is rare. It is, however, seen in cases with compensated cirrhosis.

Bimanual palpation may reveal unilateral or bilateral renal enlargement, so polycystic kidney disease must be considered. Renal bruits suggestive of renal artery stenosis may be heard 10 cm lateral and 5 cm above the umbilicus, although they are often better heard by listening in the back.

The central nervous system

Examination may reveal evidence of neurological defect due to cerebrovascular disease.

The optic fundi

Ophthalmoscopy is an integral part of the assessment of every hypertensive patient with a diastolic blood pressure greater than 110 mmHg, diabetes mellitus or renal failure. A good view must be obtained, if necessary in a darkened room, with dilatation of the pupils by tropicamide eye drops. The most frequent findings in hypertensives are:

Increased arterial tortuosity This physical sign is as much related to the age of the patient as to the height of the blood pressure.

Silver wire changes In the retinal arteries, silver wire change suggests arteriolar wall thickening. It is seen in hypertensive patients, but also occurs with advancing age.

Arteriovenous nipping or nicking Arteriovenous nipping occurs when the

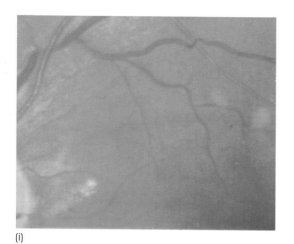

(i)

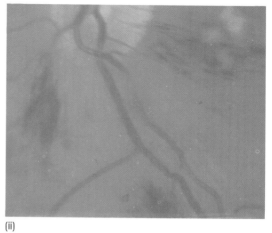

(ii)

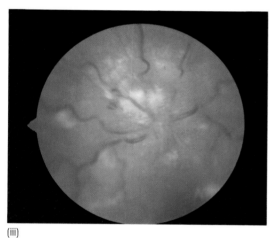

(iii)

Figure 7.4

Optic changes in hypertension. (i) Cotton wool spots and arteriovenous nipping. (ii) Cotton wool spots and flame–shaped haemorrhages. (iii) Retinal haemorrhages, exudates and papilloedema.

retinal veins appear to be narrowed or occluded as they pass under the thickened retinal arteries.

However, all of these changes can occur in normotensive subjects, particularly as they become older. The important findings in the retina that suggest severe hypertension requiring immediate action are shown in Fig. 7.4.

Retinal flame-shaped haemorrhages These are related to malignant hypertension or retinal vein occlusion.

Soft fluffy exudates or cotton wool spots These are now know to be retinal infarcts.

Hard shiny exudates These are lipid-laden retinal infarcts that frequently radiate from the macula (macula star).

Papilloedema Swelling of the optic disc. This is usually associated with raised intracranial pressure or ischaemic optic neuropathy caused by malignant hypertension. It is occasionally seen in malignant hypertension in the absence of retinal haemorrhages or exudates.

If any of the above are seen, this is a medical emergency and blood pressure must be treated promptly.

The Keith, Wagener and Barker classification of hypertensive retinopathy (below) is out of date and is misleading in that Grades III and IV are changes that occur in accelerated or malignant phase hypertension, and there is no point in differentiating between them as they have the same implications and prognosis.

- Grade I Minor vessel change only.
- Grade II Silver wire vessel change, arterial tortuosity and arteriovenous nipping.
- Grade III Retinal haemorrhages and/or cotton wool spots and/or shiny hard exudates with no papilloedema.
- Grade IV Retinal haemorrhages, exudates with papilloedema.

This classification is frequently referred to in medical journals and textbooks, but it is better simply to document the actual features seen.

Other types of retinopathy

Diabetic retinopathy may be present in hypertensive diabetics. It is particularly associated with poor control of blood pressure, inadequate control of blood sugar, longstanding diabetes and possibly cigarette smoking. If there is evidence of new vessel formation, i.e. proliferative retinopathy, patients should be referred immediately to an ophthalmologist for photocoagulation therapy.

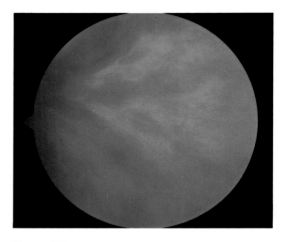

Figure 7.5
Central retinal vein thrombosis.

Unilateral retinal vein thrombosis or branch vein thrombosis with multiple haemorrhages occurs more commonly in hypertensive patients (Fig. 7.5). Retinal artery occlusion with ischaemic pallor and empty arteries is also associated with hypertension, and can be precipitated in accelerated hypertension by too rapid lowering of the blood pressure.

INVESTIGATIONS

Renal investigations

Urinalysis The urine should be tested with dipsticks at least once in all newly diagnosed hypertensive patients and thereafter at least annually. Severe hypertensive patients with or without renal disease should have their urine tested at each visit to the clinic.

Proteinuria Proteinuria can occur both in malignant hypertension, where it is due to fibrinoid necrosis, and in the non-malignant phase, due to hypertensive nephrosclerosis. If proteinuria is heavy, however, it suggests a diagnosis of intrinsic renal disease, for example, glomerulonephritis or nephrotic syndrome. Dipstick tests for urinary protein are now very sensitive, becoming positive when urinary protein is above 300 mg/l. If proteinuria is persistent this should be further investigated by a 24-hour urine collection.

Haematuria This occurs in many intrinsic renal conditions associated with hypertension, including renal cancer, glomerulonephritis or pyelonephritis, as well as various urological conditions, all of which need thorough investigation. Haematuria is common in malignant and non-malignant hypertension.

Glycosuria Glycosuria suggests the diagnosis of diabetes mellitus (see Chapter 14). Furthermore, diuretics (particularly thiazides) used in treating hypertension are diabetogenic.

Urine microscopy and culture

This is not a useful routine investigation. It should be reserved for patients who have urinary symptoms or those in whom urine dipsticks have revealed an abnormality. Reliable contaminant-free midstream specimens of urine are hard to obtain and are time-consuming for bacteriological laboratories. Bacterial growth without leucocytes is not an indicator of urinary infection. However, the presence of leucocytes in the urine without bacterial growth (sterile pyuria) is an important finding and is most often due to partially treated urine infection but also occurs in renal tuberculosis or renal tumours.

Routine blood tests

All patients who require antihypertensive drugs should also undergo routine biochemical and haematological profiling, although in most cases no abnormalities will be found.

Haematology

Polycythaemia Mild polycythaemia commonly occurs in essential hypertension. Frank polycythaemia occurs in some renal tumours. In population studies, haemoglobin levels and blood pressure are weakly correlated. A raised haemoglobin level should raise the possibility of Cushing's syndrome, alcohol excess and chronic chest disease.

Anaemia In the presence of chronic renal failure, there is usually a normochromic normocytic anaemia. This is due to deficient erythropoietin, bone marrow depression due to uraemia, mild haemolysis and, sometimes, intestinal blood loss.

Macrocytosis A raised MCV is a moderately reliable indicator of excessive alcohol intake. Hypertensive patients who have MCVs greater than 95 fl should be carefully re-questioned about their drinking habits.

Plasma viscosity or ESR These tests are very non-specific, but if they are raised then the possibility of a vasculitic disease should be considered. Both polyarteritis nodosa and systemic lupus erythematosus are associated with hypertension (see Chapter 14).

Biochemistry

Plasma sodium Plasma sodium is high or high/normal in primary hyperaldosteronism (142–150 mmol/l) and returns to normal with treatment with spironolactone or with surgery.

In renal or malignant hypertension, with or without chronic renal failure, there may be secondary hyperaldosteronism but in this situation serum sodium is low or low/normal (125–138 mmol/l). Diuretics can also cause a low plasma sodium, which may occasionally be profound.

Plasma potassium The commonest cause of hypokalaemia is diuretic therapy. In the absence of diuretic therapy, a serum potassium of 3.5 mmol/1 or less is a strong indicator of either primary or secondary aldosterone excess and always requires further investigation.

Hyperkalaemia occurs in acute renal failure but it may also occur if potassium-sparing diuretics are given to patients with renal failure, particularly if given with potassium supplementation. Hypokalaemia may develop when potassium-sparing diuretics are given together with ACE inhibitors.

Plasma bicarbonate Hypokalaemia, due to excess aldosterone, causes a metabolic alkalosis with a high plasma bicarbonate. A metabolic acidosis with low serum bicarbonate in association with hypokalaemia suggests renal tubular disease, particularly renal tubular acidosis.

Blood urea or creatinine Plasma creatinine is a less labile index of renal function than blood urea. Patients should have their renal function monitored regularly, at least once a year, even if previous results are normal. In cases with chronic renal failure, plotting serial measurements of serum creatinine on a reciprocal creatinine chart (Fig 7.6) can be a useful guide to predict the likely onset of end-stage renal disease. Estimations of creatinine clearance are not particularly useful in the routine management of hypertension.

Plasma creatinine should be checked routinely within a few weeks of starting ACE inhibitor therapy. If the creatinine rises significantly then a diagnosis of renal artery stenosis should be considered.

Serum calcium Hypertension is present in up to 60% of cases of primary hyperthyroidism. Thiazide diuretics can also cause mild rises in plasma calcium and may reveal covert primary hyperparathyroidism.

Serum phosphate A raised serum phosphate occurs in chronic renal failure, whereas in primary hyperparathyroidism low levels are seen.

Plasma uric acid Hyperuricaemia is found in about 40% of untreated patients with essential hypertension, even when renal function is normal. It is more common when hypertension is associated with renal damage. Hyperuricaemia is also common in people who consume excess alcohol. Diuretic therapy causes serum uric acid to be raised in 60% of cases even though clinical gout is seen much less commonly (about 2%).

Serum lipids The height of the serum cholesterol is an important independent predictor of coronary heart disease (see Chapter 2). There is also an association

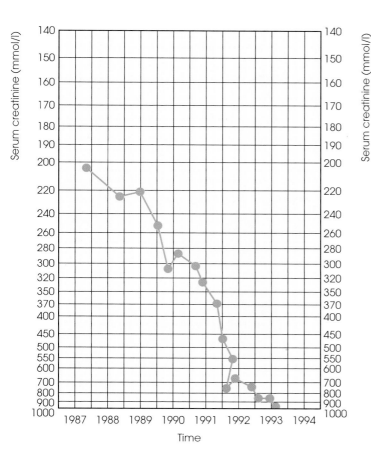

Figure 7.6
Example of a reciprocal creatinine chart in a patient with progressive chronic renal failure.

between hypercholesterolaemia and hypertension. All hypertensive patients should have a random cholesterol measurement. If this is raised, fasting cholesterol and triglyceride levels should be measured, together with either LDL or HDL cholesterol.

Gamma glutamyl transferase (γGT) or aspartate aminotransferase These enzymes are useful indicators of liver damage that may be related to alcohol excess.

Thyroid function tests Many patients may develop subclinical hypothyroidism, and T_4 and TSH levels should be measured where there is any suspicion of thyroid disease.

Chest X-ray

Radiological assessment of cardiac size is not reliable as variations occur depending on the depth of inspiration. For this reason a chest

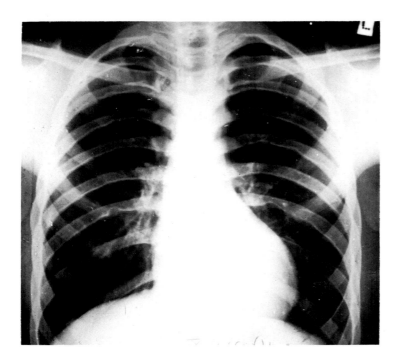

Figure 7.7
X–ray of a patient with aortic coarctation showing notching of the inferior surfaces of the third to seventh ribs.

x-ray may be omitted unless specifically indicated. It is necessary if there is concurrent chest disease or left ventricular failure. The cardiothoracic ratio (CTR) should be requested each time a chest x-ray is taken.

The presence of fractured ribs should raise the possibility of alcohol excess.

In coarctation of the aorta there is notching of the inferior edge of the second to sixth ribs owing to the dilated intercostal arteries (Fig. 7.7). There may also be sharp indentation of the lateral border of the initial portion of the descending aorta (The figure 3 sign).

Electrocardiogram

All hypertensive patients should have an ECG. It is particularly useful as a reference if the patient subsequently develops symptoms of coronary heart disease. Ideally all severe hypertensive patients should have an ECG annually; it may reveal evidence of myocardial infarction or LVH. The ECG abnormalities in LVH are:

(a) Biphasic p wave in leads V1 and V2 indicating left atrial dilatation. This is not a very specific ECG sign.
(b) Tall R waves (more than 12 mm) in a lead aVF.
(c) Chest lead criteria: The sum of the R wave in V5 or V6 with the S wave in V1 when greater than 35 mm strongly suggests the presence of LVH. These are the Solokow and Lyon criteria, which are most commonly used in clinical practice
(d) ST depression and T wave inversion in leads V5 and V6 indicate relative

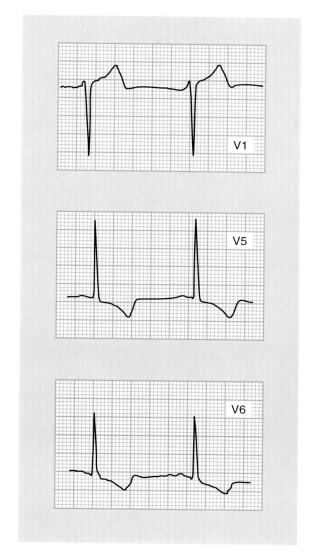

Figure 7.8

The Sokolow and Lyon measurement to assess left ventricular hypertrophy (LVH). In this example, $SV_1 = 19$ and $RV_5 = 21$: total 40 mm indicating severe LVH. Note also the ST/T changes of "strain".

ischaemia due to a hypertrophied left ventricle (the so-called strain' pattern).

When there is severe LVH, the chest lead voltages may be so large that they cannot be recorded on the narrow ECG paper. Under these circumstances, the ECG technician may reduce the voltage from 10 to 5 mm/mV. The leads are then labelled V1/2 to V6/2 with the appropriate calibration marks.

The ECG criteria for LVH are relatively crude and may miss many patients who have hypertrophy. Echocardiography is better but not always available (see Chapter 8). Nevertheless, if present, LVH does indicate that the hypertension is sustained and should be treated assiduously, as the risk of death for a given level of blood pressure is three times greater in these patients compared with those with the same pressure but no LVH (Fig. 7.8).

Twenty-four hour urinary sodium

With the increasing awareness of the value of sodium restriction in the treatment of hypertension, there is a good case for measuring 24-hour urinary sodium and potassium excretion at the first assessment, and thereafter to monitor the reduction of salt intake in the diet. Many patients claim not to be eating large amounts of salt and are often surprised by the amounts of sodium excreted in their 24-hour urine collections. This is because much of the salt they consume is hidden in processed or convenience foods.

INVESTIGATION OF HYPERTENSION IN PRIMARY CARE

The investigation of hypertension in primary care is discussed in Chapter 13. For the primary care practitioner, a reasonable rule is to investigate all patients in whom drug treatment is thought necessary. The investigations needed are a urine test, a biochemical profile including cholesterol and an ECG.

No abnormalities will be found in most patients, but when they are, they are usually important. More detailed investigation, possibly with referral to a unit with a special interest in high blood pressure, should be

reserved for those who fulfil the following criteria:

1. Clinical suspicion of an underlying cause of hypertension.
2. Moderate to severe hypertension.
3. Young (less than 35 years old).
4. Raised plasma creatinine.
5. Blood, protein or cells in the urine.
6. Low plasma potassium.
7. Variable blood pressure.
8. Failure to respond to treatment.
9. A large postural drop in blood pressure.

FURTHER INVESTIGATION

The more detailed investigations to be conducted in these cases are discussed in Chapter 8. In a large primary health care group, there may be one GP who specialises in hypertension who may choose to investigate further without hospital referral.

In hospital practice there are still too few clinics with a specific interest in the investigation and treatment of patients with high blood pressure. Patients often end up distributed between cardiologists, nephrologists and general physicians, and clinical care can become very unsystematic. There is a need for specialised blood pressure clinics that, in close liaison with primary medical care, can investigate hypertensive patients more logically and manage them more efficiently, with the long-term aim of achieving better control of blood pressure.

FURTHER READING

Berglund C, Anderson O, Wilhelmsen L. Prevalence of primary and secondary hypertension: studies in a random population sample. *Br Med J* 1977; **2**: 554.

Gifford RW, Kirkendall W, O'Connor DT, *et al*. Office evaluation of hypertension: a statement for health professionals by a writing group of the Council for High Blood Pressure Research, American Heart Association. *Hypertension* 1989; **13**: 283–93.

Harvey JM, Howie AJ, Lee SJ, *et al*. Renal biopsy findings in hypertensive patients with proteinuria. *Lancet* 1992; **340**: 1435–6.

Lip GYH, Beevers M, Beevers DG. The failure of malignant hypertension to decline. A survey of 24 years experience in multiracial population in England. *J Hypertens* 1994; **12**: 1297–1305.

Moser M. Can the cost of care be contained and quality of care maintained in the management of hypertension? *Arch Intern Med* 1994; **154**: 1665–72.

Semple PF. ABC of blood pressure management. Investigation. *Br Med J* 1981; **282**: 1306–9.

8 FURTHER INVESTIGATION OF HYPERTENSION

BACKGROUND

Hypertension is very common, with approximately 10% of the population having persistently raised blood pressure on repeated measurement. The majority of these people have essential hypertension. Patients with an underlying cause of their hypertension are relatively rare, and tend to be underinvestigated. However, this trend is changing with improved diagnostic tests and more sophisticated treatment. Many patients with secondary hypertension can now be cured, or treated more appropriately. Therefore, it is important when treating hypertension always to bear in mind the possibility of an underlying renal or adrenal disease. This chapter outlines the types of tests that can be done and the more important causes of secondary hypertension.

HOW FAR TO INVESTIGATE

The routine tests described in the previous chapter may point to there being an underlying renal or adrenal condition causing the hypertension. However, some of these underlying causes, for example phaeochromocytoma or renal artery stenosis, may be missed unless more detailed investigations are carried out. The clinician is therefore faced with a dilemma on how far to investigate, bearing in mind the costs of the tests and the very low yield if they are performed on all patients.

In Chapter 7 we listed nine criteria for further investigation, and most of those are based on particular clinical symptoms and signs, or abnormalities detected by routine tests. More detailed tests should also be done on patients who are young or have severe hypertension and on those whose blood pressures are proving difficult to control.

BRIEF DESCRIPTION OF FURTHER TESTS

Renal ultrasound

A simple non-invasive test, renal ultrasound is very useful for looking at renal size and detecting renal scarring, cysts or ureteric obstruction. It may also pick up adrenal masses as well as other abnormalities in the abdomen, including abdominal aortic aneurysm but it does not always exclude them.

In renal artery stenosis, ultrasound may demonstrate a difference in renal size. However, a lack of difference in size does not exclude this diagnosis. This cannot therefore be regarded as a suitable screening test for renovascular disease.

Plain x-ray of the abdomen

This is rarely done, but a plain x-ray of the abdomen may reveal unsuspected renal or vascular calcification, renal stones or occasionally a difference in kidney size. Phaeochromocytomas may occasionally be seen as a soft tissue shadow above one kidney.

Intravenous urography

Once considered a routine investigation in patients referred to hospital with high blood pressure, intravenous urography (IVU) is time-consuming and, occasionally, may produce life-threatening allergic reactions. It has now fallen out of favour, particularly with the advent of angiography using much smaller catheters and digital subtraction techniques. An IVU is only now appropriate for the investigation of haematuria. It is not reliable for pyelonephritis or glomerulonephritis. In our view it is not a useful screening test for renovascular hypertension as the classical features of a delayed nephrogram and later hyperconcentration may be absent.

Renal angiogram

The renal angiogram is the only test that can exclude renal artery stenosis. With modern techniques the procedure can be done on a day-patient basis and has only a slightly higher incidence of problems than the IVU, because of arterial catheterisation. Very clear anatomical pictures of the renal arteries are obtained.

In patients with renal impairment, even the much smaller amounts of contrast that are now given may cause a deterioration in renal function. It is extremely important that patients are well hydrated before the angiogram.

Radioisotope imaging

Radioisotope renograms are used in the diagnosis of renal artery stenosis, often before and after an ACE inhibitor, usually captopril. There is considerable controversy about the ability of this test to exclude renal artery stenosis. It is certainly useful as a follow-up procedure in patients with renal artery stenosis following angioplasty or surgery.

A radio-labelled analogue of guanethidine, metaiodobenzyl guanidine (MIBG), is concentrated in some phaeochromocytomas and this is a useful test in conjunction with CT scanning, particularly when there are multiple or extra-adrenal tumours. However, some tumours do not take up the isotope and too much reliance should not be placed on the test, particularly when it is negative.

Selenium cholesterol scans of the adrenal gland have also been used to detect aldosterone-secreting adrenal adenomas, as cholesterol is taken up by some of these tumours. However, our experience is that the test is often not helpful and may be misleading. It is much better to rely on CT or MRI scans (see primary aldosteronism later in the chapter).

CT and MRI scans

CT scans have revolutionised the investigation of adrenal causes of hypertension and are particularly useful in localising phaeochromocytomas and adrenal adenomas secreting aldosterone. However, both scans are expensive. They should only be carried out if there is biochemical evidence of aldosterone or catecholamine excess, or some other indication.

MRI scanning may occasionally be more useful if CT scans have provided equivocal results when localising adrenal adenomas.

Echocardiography

Echocardiography is a more accurate method of assessing left ventricular size and wall thickness than the ECG. Where available, it is a useful test, particularly in assessing patients with borderline hypertension or who are suspected of having 'white-coat hypertension' where the finding of left ventricular hypertrophy (LVH) may indicate that the blood pressure level is more sustained. It may also be useful in the follow-up of patients who have enlargement of the left ventricle to see whether hypertrophy regresses as blood pressure is controlled.

Abnormalities of left ventricular systolic function may also be detected before the onset of clinical evidence of cardiac failure.

Twenty-four-hour urine collections

An accurate collection of 24-hour urine is vital to avoid misleading results, particularly for catecholamine collections. It is therefore very important that the correct procedure is explained to the patient, and that a large enough bottle or three 1-litre bottles are provided together with a non-transparent carrier bag. It helps to give printed instructions to the patient or have instructions written on the side of the bottle. However, in our experience, it is best if a nurse also goes through the instructions in detail as often patients have difficulties in understanding exactly what is required (Table 8.1).

Sodium and potassium

Nearly all the sodium and most of the potassium we eat comes out in the urine, so a 24-hour collection is a good guide to intake. The test is therefore useful in trying to find out how much salt is consumed and whether patients are complying with advice about the reduction of salt intake.

Catecholamine excretion

The measurement of urinary metabolites of adrenaline (epinephrine) and noradrenaline (norepinephrine) or their metabolites is the best screening test for the rare but curable phaeochromocytoma. Depending on the local laboratory, different metabolites of catecholamines are measured. Urinary metanephrines and vanillylmandelic acid (VMA) are the most commonly assayed. However, probably the best measurement, where available, is the excretion of urinary noradrenaline and adrenaline. It is very important for these hormonal measurements that the urine collection is an exact one and contains sufficient hydrochloric acid to preserve the catecholamine. Patients should be warned that the acid can cause skin burns until it has been diluted with urine.

For the Guidance of Patients

24-HOUR URINE COLLECTION

1. It is *IMPORTANT* to collect all urine that your kidneys make during a 24-hour period.
2. The collection should start in the morning between 6.00 a.m. and 10.00 a.m. The exact time you start should be written down.
3. For example, if you start on Sunday at 6.00 a.m. then you should finish your collection at 6.00 a.m. on Monday.
4. When you start the collection, empty your bladder and discard the urine.
5. All urine produced for the next 24 hours should be put in the bottle provided.
6. Exactly 24 hours after starting a collection, empty bladder whether you need to or not, but this time into the bottle.

If you forget or spill some of your urine during this period the collection is no good. Discard the urine and collect a new bottle from the laboratory or the Out-Patients Department.

HINTS

1. Put the bottle in the toilet so that you do not forget to use it.
2. Ladies may find it easier to pass urine into a jug and then put it into a bottle.
3. When you find the need to open your bowels, make sure you pass urine into the bottle first.

IMPORTANT

The 24-hour specimen of urine must be brought into the hospital on the same day it is completed.

Table 8.1
An example of instructions for patients to obtain an accurate 24-hour urine collection.

Creatinine excretion

Measurement of creatinine excretion is useful to assess the completeness of a 24-hour urine collection as the average creatinine excretion is around 1 g/day. It will be more in men and particularly those with a large muscle bulk. If plasma creatinine is measured concurrently, a creatinine clearance can be calculated. There is no need to determine the creatinine clearance in patients whose serum creatinine is in the normal range.

When monitoring serial changes in renal function we prefer to measure serum creatinine levels only and employ a reciprocal creatinine chart (Chapter 7).

Urinary protein

If dipstick tests show more than a trace of proteinuria, a 24-hour collection should be carried out to measure total urinary protein loss. Dipsticks are only positive if the concentration of protein in the urine exceeds 300 mg/l, which is 10 times the upper limit of normal.

Microproteinuria is present when the 24-hour urine protein loss is between 30 and 300 mg/day. This finding is highly predictive of renal failure in patients with diabetes mellitus. In hypertensive patients without diabetes this test is of uncertain value.

BLOOD HORMONE MEASUREMENTS

The renin–angiotensin system

All the components of the renin–angiotensin system can be measured, but the commonest and easiest measurement is plasma renin activity. This gives the rate of formation of angiotensin I in plasma, which has been shown to correlate closely with the prevailing level of plasma angiotensin II. Plasma aldosterone can also be measured by radioimmunoassay. The tests are indicated where there is suspected renal artery stenosis or a renin-secreting tumour, where renin levels may be high. In primary aldosteronism, plasma renin activity is low and plasma aldosterone will be high due to the autonomous secretion of aldosterone from an adrenal adenoma. In secondary aldosteronism, the high levels of renin and angiotensin II are the cause of the raised aldosterone.

Plasma catecholamines

Measurement of plasma adrenaline and noradrenaline levels is helpful in the diagnosis of phaeochromocytoma, particularly during an 'attack' when there is a sudden rise in blood pressure, possibly with tachycardia and blanching. These assays are only available in a few specialist centres.

Plasma cortisol

A random plasma cortisol level may occasionally be useful in the diagnosis of Cushings disease. However, if the index of suspicion is high it is best to measure the diurnal rhythm of plasma cortisol or proceed to a dexamethsone suppression test.

ADRENAL CAUSES OF HIGH BLOOD PRESSURE

Primary aldosteronism

This syndrome is due to excessive secretion of aldosterone by the adrenal gland. This causes sodium and water retention with suppression of the renin system leading to low levels of plasma renin activity. There are two major causes of primary aldosteronism. The first is due to a small 0.5–2 cm benign adenoma of the adrenal cortex, which is directly responsible for the high levels of aldosterone. When the adenoma is removed the condition is usually cured or greatly improved. The other cause of primary aldosteronism is bilateral adrenal hyperplasia, where both adrenal glands oversecrete aldosterone due to mechanisms that are not fully understood. Again there is sodium and water retention and suppression of the renin–angiotensin system. These patients present with a similar clinical and biochemical picture with sodium and water retention, moderately raised plasma sodium levels, high blood pressure, reduced plasma potassium concentrations, and inappropriately high potassium excretion.

These two conditions need to be distinguished from secondary aldosteronism, where high aldosterone levels are elevated due to raised renin release and angiotensin II formation. This occurs in as malignant hypertension, renal artery stenosis and where there is sodium and water depletion usually due to diuretic treatment. In this situation, plasma potassium will also be low, but it is relatively easy to distinguish primary and secondary aldosteronism because the plasma renin activity is high in secondary aldosteronism, and low in primary aldosteronism. It is vital, therefore, when measuring plasma aldosterone levels to also measure plasma renin activity.

Clinical features

Most patients with primary aldosteronism (Conn's Syndrome) have high blood pressure and low plasma potassium levels, although in the early stages, particularly in patients who restrict salt intake, plasma potassium may not be low. In some patients, particularly those with a high salt intake, potassium levels may be very low and they may present with muscle weakness, tiredness and arrhythmias. This is particularly likely to happen if thiazide diuretics are given, as this causes a further fall in plasma potassium. Patients with primary aldosteronism can, contrary to some reports, develop malignant or accelerated hypertension. Any patient who develops hypokalaemia whilst receiving a low dose of a thiazide diuretic should be investigated in detail to exclude a diagnosis of Conn's Syndrome.

Biochemical features

The hallmark of primary aldosteronism is a low plasma potassium, i.e. below 3.4 mmol/l, combined with a raised plasma sodium concentration (usually to between 140 and 150 mmol/l) and a metabolic alkalosis, with an increase in plasma bicarbonate levels. The 24-hour excretion of potassium will also be inappropriately high for the low plasma potassium levels. Plasma

aldosterone levels will be high with a low plasma renin activity. Ideally, these measurements should be done when patients are not receiving drug treatment, with a concomitant 24-hour urine collection to assess salt intake. However, in many patients this may be unnecessary as the ratio of plasma aldosterone levels to plasma renin activity is a good index of aldosterone excess.

More complicated tests used to be done to distinguish between adenomas and bilateral hyperplasia. In general, patients with adenomas have a loss of diurnal variation of plasma aldosterone, and aldosterone suppression does not occur after salt loading or fludrocortisone. These tests are now rarely done since the advent of CT or MRI scanning.

CT and MRI scans

CT and MRI scanning have revolutionised the investigation of primary aldosteronism. Most adenomas can be detected if they are greater than 0.5 cm in diameter by high quality resolution CT scans (Fig. 8.1).

Adrenal venography and adrenal vein sampling

Before CT scanning became available, adrenal venography and adrenal vein sampling were necessary to locate adrenal adenomas. These investigations are hazardous as they may lead to adrenal infarction. The only indication at present is when there is some doubt as to whether there is an adenoma. Even here, in our view, it is better in patients with negative CT scans to treat their blood pressure with spironolactone and repeat the CT scan at

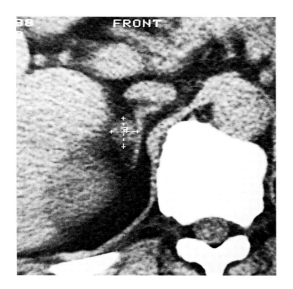

Figure 8.1
CT scan showing a large right adrenal tumour which was an aldosterone-secreting adenoma.

2–3 year intervals. If they have an adrenal adenoma it will eventually become larger and will then be visible on the CT scan.

Treatment

Once the adrenal adenoma has been localised it is usual to remove it (Fig. 8.2). Conventionally, this required a major abdominal operation, but it is now possible to remove the adrenal through a loin incision or by a 'laparoscopic' technique. Now that surgery is less hazardous, more patients can benefit from the procedure. In cases where surgery is not feasible, the aldosterone antagonist, spironolactone, may be given. Conventionally, high doses were given (100–300 mg/day), which usually caused side-effects. However, lower doses of spironolactone are effective, particularly when combined with other drugs.

With removal of the adenoma, plasma potassium invariably returns to normal; however, blood pressure does not always return to normal although it may be greatly improved. It is important that this is explained to patients before an operation as they may be disappointed to find they still need some drug therapy afterwards.

In rare cases, carcinoma of the adrenal gland may secrete excessive aldosterone levels, and it is important to bear this in

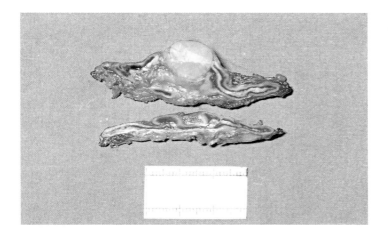

Figure 8.2
Typical adrenal adenoma causing primary aldosteronism.

mind when assessing the need for surgery. Aldosterone-secreting carcinomas are usually large (≥ 3 cm) and the patients are clinically unwell due to oversecretion of other hormones.

Bilateral adrenal hyperplasia

The biochemical features in patients with bilateral hyperplasia are similar to those with adenomas but no tumour is found. Both the adrenal glands are hypertrophied and, as yet, there is no specific treatment for this condition and the aetiology is unknown. Blood pressure may be resistant to treatment. Usually a potassium-conserving diuretic such as spironolactone or amiloride will correct the hypokalaemia, and calcium-channel blockers may be effective when combined with the diuretic. Salt restriction is useful in controlling blood pressure as well as in correcting hypokalaemia.

It should always be borne in mind that these patients could have a very small adenoma not detected even by high-resolution CT scanning, and as there is now evidence that some patients with bilateral hyperplasia

may subsequently be found to have an adrenal adenoma, so reassessment every few years is necessary.

Rarely, a familial form of hyperaldosteronism may be found, which can be controlled with dexamethasone. Patients with any suggestion of a family history of hypertension, premature strokes and low serum potassium levels should be referred to a specialist centre for further investigation.

Other causes of hypokalaemia

The finding of a low plasma potassium in hypertensive patients is relatively common, so it is important to exclude other causes before assuming that it is due to primary aldosteronism (Table 8.2). The commonest cause of hypokalaemia is the use of high doses of thiazide diuretics. Serum potassium levels may remain low for up to 4 weeks after treatment has been stopped. A low plasma potassium also occurs with intestinal potassium loss, particularly where there is chronic vomiting, usually surreptitious, or chronic diarrhoea for example due to laxative abuse.

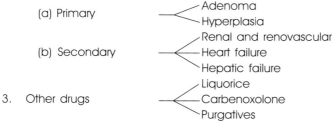

1. Diuretic therapy in high dose
2. Aldosteronism

    (a) Primary   Adenoma / Hyperplasia

    (b) Secondary   Renal and renovascular / Heart failure / Hepatic failure

3. Other drugs   Liquorice / Carbenoxolone / Purgatives

4. Congenital renal tubular acidosis

Table 8.2
Causes of hypokalaemia with high blood pressure.

Carbenoxolone therapy and liquorice ingestion cause an electrolyte picture identical to that occurring in primary aldosteronism (see Chapter 5), so it is important to question patients about their liquorice intake. Patients with very high plasma renin levels that may occur in malignant and renovascular hypertension may have hypokalaemia, but usually the plasma sodium concentration is also low, whereas in primary aldosteronism, sodium levels are usually raised. Secondary aldosterone excess can also occur in heart failure and in hepatic disease.

Rarely, renal tubular defects can cause excessive loss of urinary potassium. This is associated with failure to acidify the urine and a metabolic acidosis with renal stones. Blood pressure is usually normal.

Cushing's syndrome

Cushing's syndrome results from excessive secretion of cortisol, which may be either due to autonomous oversecretion by the adrenal gland or to raised ACTH levels from a pituitary tumour. Cushing's syndrome is usually suspected on the basis of the patient's clinical appearance. The diagnosis is confirmed by an overnight dexamethasone suppression test. Some lung tumours may also secrete ACTH and cause excess cortisol and aldosterone secretion. These patients present with low potassium levels and high blood pressure, not unlike primary aldosteronism. Further investigations to distinguish between ACTH-secreting tumours and excessive cortisol secretion by adrenal tumours or hyperplasia involve a variety of specialised endocrine tests.

Alcoholism may occasionally cause a clinical and biochemical picture similar to Cushing's syndrome and it is worthwhile checking liver enzymes, particularly gamma glutamyl transferase in patients with suspected Cushing's syndrome.

Adrenal enzyme deficiencies

Various congenital deficiencies of the enzymes responsible for the synthesis of adrenal steroids from the precursor cholesterol have been described. Most of these deficiencies present early in childhood, the commonest presenting with virilisation. Only two of them are associated with high blood pressure, that is 11–alpha and 17–beta hydroxylase deficiency, which are associated with the production of large amounts of mineralocorticoid hormones. These patients need highly specialised investigation in a paediatric endocrinology unit.

Occasionally there may be partial enzyme defects that may not be picked up until adulthood.

Whether subtle abnormalities of adrenal enzyme activity are responsible for the elevation of blood pressure in some patients with essential hypertension remains a matter of controversy.

Phaeochromocytoma

These chromaffin cell tumours produce the most dramatic form of secondary hypertension. They are usually found in the adrenal medulla but may occur in the sympathetic chain, particularly in the retroperitoneal space. They have also been described in the thoracic sympathetic chain and in many other parts of the body. They are characterised by intermittent or continuous oversecretion of noradrenaline and adrenaline, which causes the symptoms of tachycardia, blanching, sweating and sudden rises in blood pressure.

These tumours may present at any age and are not uncommon in children. Most patients have severe hypertension, often in the malignant phase. However, in some patients, blood pressure may only be mildly raised and there may be intermittent surges of high blood pressure associated with release of the catecholamines. Some patients may present with postural hypotension (Table 8.3).

Table 8.3
Clinical features of phaeochromocytoma

Blood pressure

Hypertension 98%	–	intermittent	30%
	–	sustained	50%
	–	paroxysmal	20%
	–	malignant phase	40%
Persistently normotensive 2%			

Site

Abdominal	98%
– adrenal	70%
– extra-adrenal	10%
– multiple	20%
– bilateral	10%
Thoracic	2%
Neck	<1%
Familial	10%
Malignant tumour	10%

Symptoms

Headache	80%
Sweating	70%
Palpitations	60%
Nervousness	40%
Nausea	40%
Weight loss	40%

Diagnosis

While phaeochromocytomas are very rare, the outlook for a patient with the disease is extremely poor as fatal hypertensive crises may occur during anaesthesia, pregnancy and other stresses. Occasionally the diagnosis is not made until autopsy. The only way of diagnosing phaeochromocytoma is by the measurement of urinary metabolites and/or plasma noradrenaline and adrenaline levels. It is not feasible to screen all hypertensive patients with these measurements, so clinical acumen has to be used in selecting those patients needing further investigations. The following features suggest the need for measurement of catecholamines levels:

- A story of intermittent high blood pressure, sweating attacks and palpitations.
- Patients presenting with weight loss and high blood pressure, particularly if there is associated postural hypotension.
- All patients with resistant or malignant phase hypertension.
- Hypertensive patients diagnosed below age 35 years.

Investigation

The simplest investigation is a 24-hour urine collection for measurement of the catecholamines themselves or their metabolites, for example vanillylmandelic acid (VMA) or the metanephrines. However, occasionally VMA or metanephrines may be normal. The measurement of urinary noradrenaline, adrenaline and dopamine may be a better method of screening patients, if available. Plasma noradrenaline and adrenaline levels are raised in most patients with phaeochromocytoma but may

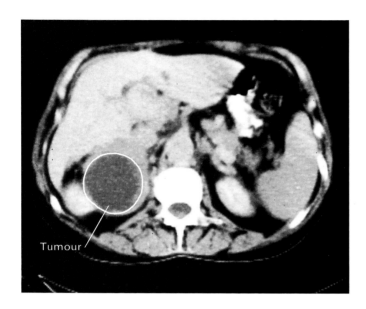

Tumour

Figure 8.3
CT scan of a large right adrenal
phaeochromyocytoma.

also be normal, particularly if there are intermittent surges of noradrenaline and
adrenaline release.

If the urinary or plasma catecholamines
are raised, abdominal ultrasound may locate
the tumours, although CT scanning is the
most accurate technique (Fig. 8.3). The
majority of the tumours are in the adrenal
glands but they may be bilateral or extra-
adrenal and are occasionally multiple. Some
tumours, whilst histologically identical to
others, may spread locally and eventually
metastasise, particularly to the long bones
and the vertebrae. Scanning with the
radioisotope MIBG which is taken up by
some phaeochromocytomas is useful, particularly in localising extra-adrenal tumours. In
patients where there is difficulty in locating
the tumour, venous sampling from multiple
sites down the inferior vena cava may be
necessary.

Treatment

All patients with phaeochromocytomas must
have them removed (Fig. 8.4). Prior to
surgery it is very important that their blood
pressure is controlled, as during surgery
dangerous rises in blood pressure may
occur, particularly during induction of anaesthesia and when the tumour is being
mobilised prior to removal. It is vital that all
patients are very carefully prepared preop-
eratively and that the removal of the tumour
is done by an expert anaesthetic/surgical
team.

Before surgery all patients should be
treated medically. Acute paroxysms of high
blood pressure can be controlled with the
alpha-blocker phentolamine, 2–5 mg being
given intravenously or by infusion. However,
this is a short acting alpha-blocker lasting for
only a few minutes. The oral drug of choice

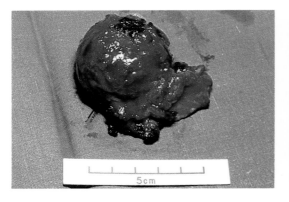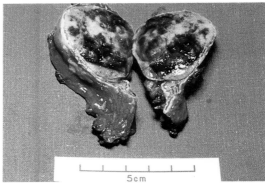

Figure 8.4
A typical phaeochromocytoma.

is phenoxybenzamine, a longer acting alpha-blocker that can be given once or twice daily. The dose should be started at 5 or 10 mg twice daily and increased until the blood pressure is controlled. Often these patients are volume-depleted and with the control of blood pressure they may develop postural hypotension. In this situation it is important to correct the deficit in sodium balance by giving extra sodium and water either orally or by intravenous infusion. A beta-blocker such as propranolol or atenolol should also be used in small doses to control the heart rate, but should not be started until the alpha-blocker has been established. This is because beta-blockade alone can sometimes cause dangerous rises in blood pressure or precipitate heart failure. Labetolol has been claimed to be of use but in our experience it is not as good as the combination of phenoxybenzamine and a beta-blocker.

It is very important that all patients are adequately alpha-blocked. Indeed, if anything, they should be slightly overtreated to overcome the intense vasoconstriction that occurs as large amounts of the catecholamines are released when the tumour is mobilised with major fluctuations in blood pressure. Once the tumour is removed, there may be profound hypotension if the patient is not adequately alpha-blocked prior to surgery. Intra-arterial blood pressure must be monitored and, if blood pressure is not controlled by the pre-operative phenoxybenzamine, either phentolamine or sodium nitroprusside should be used during surgery. Pulse rate can be controlled by an intravenous beta-blocker. At the time that the blood vessels supplying the tumour are ligated, large amounts of blood and saline may need to be given to overcome hypotension.

While most patients have a single adrenal tumour and removal cures them, phaeochromocytomas can recur, so all such patients should be followed up carefully with annual re-checking of blood or urinary catecholamines.

Rare familial varieties of phaeochromocytoma also occur, particularly in association with other endocrine tumours, most notably parathyroid adenomas and medullary cell carcinoma of the thyroid (Sipple syndrome). Phaeochromocytomas are also associated with Von Recklinghausen's neurofibromatosis and carotid body tumours. Occasionally they may occur around the renal artery, mimicking renal artery stenosis. A family history must always be obtained, and relatives should be screened.

Other neural crest tumours

Neuroblastomas and ganglioneuromas can cause hypertension with abdominal tumours. These usually occur only in children.

Hyperparathyroidism

Roughly 50% of patients with primary hyperparathyroidism have high blood pressure. The mechanism is not known and removal of the parathyroid adenoma does not usually correct the high blood pressure. Hyperparathyroidism is usually discovered on routine measurement of plasma calcium and this should be measured in all patients with hypertension. High blood pressure itself is not necessarily an indication for parathyroidectomy unless there is renal damage, metabolic bone disease or other symptoms. Thiazide diuretics themselves can cause a small increase in plasma calcium and this may reveal some patients with mild hyperparathyroidism.

Thyroid disease

Patients with hyperthyroidism often have a widened pulse pressure and a raised systolic blood pressure. Control of the thyrotoxicosis usually results in the systolic blood pressure returning to normal.

Patients with myxoedema may also have raised blood pressure, although the mechanisms for this are not known. We recommend the measurement of TSH levels in all obese hypertensive patients, particularly if they also have raised plasma lipid levels.

Acromegaly

Hypertension occurs commonly in patients with acromegaly, and cardiovascular complications are the commonest cause of death.

Coarctation of the aorta

Usually in aortic coarctation there is narrowing of the aorta just beyond the origin of the left subclavian artery. Severe cases usually present in childhood, but less severe defects may not present until adult life. Elevated blood pressure is found above the constriction with a low blood pressure below. The mechanism of the high blood pressure would appear, at least in part, to be due to a diminished perfusion of the kidneys, causing increased renin secretion and retention of sodium and water in an attempt to maintain renal perfusion pressure. This leads to raised blood pressure in the upper part of the body. The diagnosis is usually made from the simultaneous palpation of radial and femoral or radial and posterior tibial arteries. There will be diminution in strength and delay of the pulses in the legs.

If the diagnosis of coarctation is considered likely, blood pressures should be measured in the legs. A chest x-ray may confirm the diagnosis with enlargement of the heart, dilatation of the aorta round the constriction and notching of the underside of the ribs by collateral vessels. Echocardiography, CT scanning and, if necessary, aortography can all be used to localise the lesion. Surgery is usually performed, depending on the circumstances, although recently balloon angioplasty has also been used with success.

RENAL CAUSES OF HIGH BLOOD PRESSURE

High blood pressure secondary to kidney diseases may be due to the underlying kidney damage causing sodium retention or to an inappropriate release of renin, with raised plasma levels of angiotensin II. Usually, hypertension in parenchymal renal disease is due to a combination of both these factors, although it may involve other less well understood factors.

Alternatively, the hypertension itself may have initiated the renal damage, which in turn aggravates the hypertension. It is usually not possible to be certain which was the primary event.

Renal artery stenosis

Of all the causes of hypertension, renal artery stenosis has attracted the most attention. Initially it appeared to be a rare cause of hypertension but it is now clear that it is the most common cause of secondary hypertension.

Cause

The renal arterial narrowing in patients below the age of 40, particularly if they are women, is usually due to fibromuscular hyperplasia of the renal or intra-renal arteries (Fig. 8.5). In older patients the stenosis is likely to be due to vascular disease (atheroma) (Fig. 8.6). Very rarely there may be extra-arterial compression by retroperitoneal tumours. When there is a narrowing of one artery to the kidney, the reduced renal blood flow causes increased secretion of renin and high circulating levels of plasma angiotensin II. This can directly cause the blood pressure to increase. However, the situation is often more complicated because the other kidney may become damaged, so there may be secondary retention of sodium in combination with inappropriately high renin levels for the degree of sodium balance.

Diagnosis

There are no particular clinical features of renal artery stenosis but, in general, patients tend to have more resistant hypertension and may present with the malignant phase. Renal bruits are audible in about 40% of patients. All patients, therefore, with malignant hypertension or blood pressure that is resistant to conventional therapy should be thoroughly investigated for renal artery stenosis. This condition is also particularly common in patients with atheromatous vascular disease at other sites, particularly if they are heavy cigarette smokers.

Investigations

Renal angiogram The renal angiogram is the only reliable test for renal artery stenosis. It requires catherisation of the femoral artery followed by an injection of dye into the aorta and renal arteries. In experienced hands and with digital subtraction little

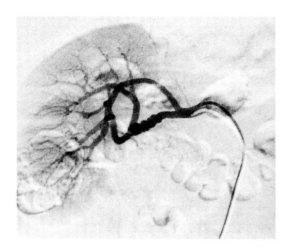

Figure 8.5

Fibromuscular hyperplasia in lower branch of renal artery.

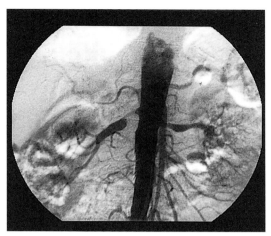

Figure 8.6

Atheromatous bilateral renal artery stenosis with post–stenotic dilatation.

contrast medium is given. Complications are rare and most patients can be investigated as day cases. In patients where other renal diseases are being looked for, it is possible to get good nephrogram pictures with the arteriogram, making intravenous pyelogram unnecessary.

Intravenous urography With the advent of simple and better angiography, IVU as a screening test for renal artery stenosis is rarely used.

Isotope renograms Renograms with and without captopril have been claimed to be a good screening test for renovascular hypertension. Our experience is that it depends on the excellence of the local nuclear medicine department, and some patients with treatable renal artery stenosis may be missed. In our view, therefore, all patients where there is a strong suspicion of renal artery stenosis should undergo renal

angiography, even if the isotope renogram is reported as normal.

Measurements of plasma renin Plasma renin levels are often raised in renal artery stenosis and there is hyper-responsiveness to various manoeuvres to stimulate renin release. However, in some patients, plasma renin levels are normal or even low, particularly where there is bilateral renal artery stenosis or a unilateral narrowing of one artery and an occluded artery on the other side.

Renal vein measurements Measuring the plasma renin activity in blood from renal veins was a widely used procedure before the advent of angioplasty, and involved catheterising both renal veins from the femoral vein. Various criteria were suggested to predict the outcome of surgery or angioplasty of the renal arteries. It was claimed that, if the renal vein renin level was at least

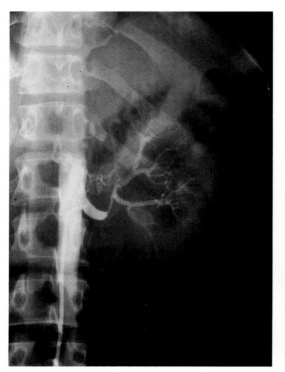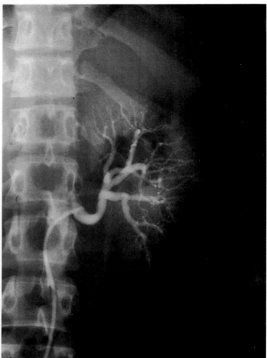

Figure 8.7
Balloon dilatation in a young woman with unilateral renal artery stenosis before (left) and after (right) angioplasty.

1.5 times higher on the affected side compared with the normal kidney, this was a strong indication of a functionally significant narrowing of the renal artery and surgical repair would be successful. However, where there is severe renal artery stenosis, blood flow to the affected kidney may be reduced and, although the kidney may be secreting very little renin, the concentration of renin in the renal vein may be high because of the reduced blood flow. When these tests are done it is important therefore to measure plasma renin activity in the vena cava, above and below the kidneys. A correction can then be made for a dimin-

ished blood flow from the affected kidney. However, there is now little need to do these measurements. Where lesions can easily be angioplastied it is probably better to do this immediately and see the effect on blood pressure rather than delaying whilst measuring the renal vein renin levels.

Treatment The advent of balloon angioplasty has changed the treatment of renal artery stenosis over the last few years (Fig. 8.7). Renal artery reconstruction is technically difficult and whether it provides any benefit over good blood pressure control with drugs remains controversial. Balloon angioplasty is a much less traumatic technique that can be successful in well-selected cases, particularly those with fibro-muscular hyperplasia. Complications such as dissection or damage to the artery or haemorrhage from the artery are rare. However, in many patients with atheroma-tous lesions, these may recur and frequent angioplasties may be necessary. In patients with more proximal stenosis of the renal arteries, particularly at the origin of the renal artery, an angioplasty may be technically difficult so it may be necessary to put a stent into the renal artery.

Well-controlled studies comparing angio-plasty to medical treatment have yielded disappointing results. However, there are many reasons why more detailed investiga-tions for renal artery stenosis are now justi-fied and angioplasty is indicated for other reasons than blood pressure control alone.

- Renal angioplasty in reliable hands can produce excellent results, particularly in younger patients with fibromuscular hyperplasia, thus avoiding lifelong drug therapy.
- Even if blood pressure is not normalised, control with drugs may be rendered easier.
- If the arterial supply to the kidney is seriously embarrassed, dilatation or opera-tion may help to preserve renal function.
- Both fibromuscular hyperplasia and atheroma are progressive diseases and might recur either in the same renal artery or on the other side.
- Some patients with hypertension and severe heart failure may have unsus-pected renal artery stenosis. Their symptoms of heart failure may improve following angioplasty.

Atheromatous renovascular disease is always associated with vascular disease elsewhere. Often patients are heavy cigarette smokers

and they should be persuaded to stop. Other steps should be taken to try and prevent the development of further progressive vascular damage. In particular, patients should reduce their cholesterol levels as much as possible. Regression of some atheromatous lesions may be possible provided patients are prepared to reduce their fat intake sufficiently and/or take cholesterol-lowering drugs. Furthermore, accurate blood pressure control is mandatory.

Renin-secreting tumours

Very rare tumours of the renal juxta-glomerular cells (haemangiopericytomas) can secrete excess renin directly causing high blood pressure. They usually occur in children or young adults who present with malignant hypertension with high levels of renin and angiotensin II and hypokalaemia secondary to the aldosterone excess. The tumours may be seen on renal angiography. If the tumour can be localised and removed, the patient may be cured.

Hypertension may also occur in children with juvenile renal tumours (Wilms' tumours), as well as in clear-cell carcinoma of the kidney in adults.

Other causes of renal hypertension

Most forms of renal disease cause high blood pressure. The only renal diseases not compli-cated by raised blood pressure are those affecting the renal medulla alone, where there may be loss of sodium and water and therefore relatively low blood pressure.

Glomerulonephritis

Both acute and chronic glomerulonephritis are associated with high blood pressure. Particularly severe hypertension may occur in patients with IgA nephropathy, very often with raised plasma renin activity. Some patients develop the malignant phase of hypertension with an acute deterioration in renal function requiring dialysis. Further investigation involves microscopy of the urine, intravenous urography, exclusion of tuberculosis by early morning urine cultures and, if indicated, a renal biopsy. Control of blood pressure is particularly important as there is increasing evidence that this can slow down the progression of many renal diseases. There is now evidence that the ACE inhibitors in particular delay the deterioration of renal function in diabetic and non-diabetic patients with nephropathy.

Pyelonephritis

The radiological features suggestive of pyelonephritis are calyceal clubbing with areas of renal cortical thinning. There remains some doubt as to whether this form of kidney damage causes hypertension unless there is associated renal failure. Similarly, there is controversy about possible associations between hypertension and chronic urinary infection. Patients with radiological evidence of pyelonephritis need detailed urological assessment to exclude obstruction of urine flow due to prostatic enlargement, pelviureteric junction (PUJ) obstruction, or pelvic tumours.

Polycystic kidney disease

An autosomal dominant condition, polycystic kidney disease causes bilateral renal cysts, berry aneurysms of the circle of Willis and, sometimes, hepatic and pancreatic cysts. Often it is not diagnosed until middle age. The presenting features are hypertension, subarachnoid haemorrhage, abdominal pain,

haematuria and, more commonly, the insidious development of renal failure. There is increasing evidence that good control of blood pressure may prevent or delay the onset of renal failure and, in particular, may also prevent subarachnoid haemorrhages. With the increasing use of ultrasound, many patients are now being picked up through screening of families, and it is important to screen all relatives of patients with polycystic kidney disease. On renal ultrasound the cysts can easily be seen (Fig. 8.8). CT scans will also clearly demonstrate the renal cysts (Fig. 8.9). Patients who are known to have polycystic kidney disease should have regular checks on their blood pressure and even very mildly elevated levels should be treated.

Diabetic kidney disease

The topic of diabetic hypertension is discussed in Chapter 14. High blood pressure is common in diabetics and is one of the best predictors of nephropathy and retinopathy. Accurate control of blood pressure is necessary, preferably with an ACE inhibitor.

CONNECTIVE TISSUE DISORDERS

Most of the connective tissue disorders can cause renal damage and are often associated with high blood pressure. Hypertension may be worsened with the use of corticosteroid therapy.

Scleroderma

Patients with scleroderma may suddenly develop malignant hypertension and acute

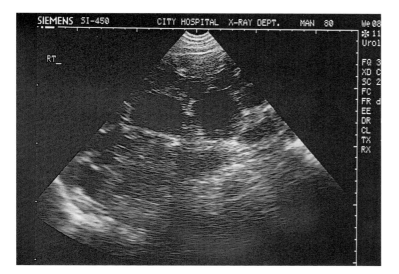

Figure 8.8
Ultrasound showing polycystic kidney.

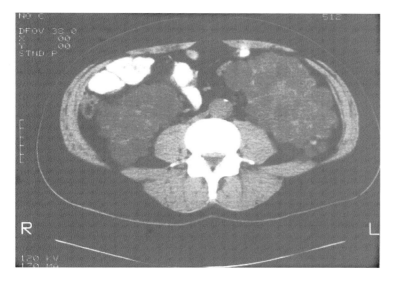

Figure 8.9
CT scan showing bilateral polycystic kidneys.

renal failure (Fig. 8.8). It is important, therefore, that blood pressure is measured and treated even if it is only mildly elevated. Some claims have been made that the ACE inhibitors may specifically prevent the development of malignant hypertension and renal failure, but whether this is correct or not is not clear. There are no diagnostic tests for scleroderma, so the diagnosis must rely on clinical criteria.

Systemic lupus erythematosus

Systemic lupus erythematosus often involves the kidney, and hypertension and renal failure are common sequelae. Corticosteroids and cytotoxic therapy may delay the progression of the renal disease. Control of blood pressure is important as a raised blood pressure may hasten the onset of renal damage. Antinuclear antibodies (ANA) and extractable nuclear antigen (ENA) may be positive. A reversible lupus-like syndrome can be caused by hydralazine therapy.

Polyarteritis nodosa

This connective tissue disorder, when it involves the kidney, can cause severe hypertension resistant to treatment. The diagnosis is made usually on other features of polyarteritis, and characteristic lesions will be seen on renal biopsy and renal angiography. Anti-neutrophil cytoplasmic antibodies (ANCA) or ANA may be positive.

Retroperitoneal fibrosis

Fibrosis of the retroperitoneal tissues may occur after treatment with methysergide, or may be associated with retroperitoneal tumours. Most often, however, no cause is found. The ureters are pulled medially and may become obstructed, causing bilateral hydronephrosis with secondary hypertension.

Obstructive uropathy

Obstructive uropathy may be associated with high blood pressure, particularly if there is renal failure. In older patients with prostatic enlargement and chronic urinary retention, high blood pressure would be expected to be common, but it appears to be no more so than in the general population of that age.

FURTHER READING

Derkx FHM, Schalekamp MADH. Renal artery stenosis and hypertension. *Lancet* 1994; **344**: 237–9.

Gonzalo A, Rivera M, Quereda C, *et al*. Clinical features and prognosis of adult polycystic kidney disease. *Am J Nephrol* 1990; **10**: 470–4.

Gordon RD. Mineralocorticoid hypertension. *Lancet* 1994; **344**: 240–3.

Raine AEG. Hypertension and the kidney. *Br Med Bull* 1994; **50**: 322–41.

Ross EJ, Griffith DNW. The clinical presentation of phaeochromocytoma. *Q J Med* 1989; **71**: 485–96.

3

Section Three

9 THE BENEFITS OF ANTIHYPERTENSIVE TREATMENT

BACKGROUND

Whilst the aetiology and pathogenesis of hypertension remain uncertain and the optimum method of reducing blood pressure is still controversial, there is no doubt that the value of antihypertensive treatment is proven. These drugs can be regarded as having benefits that rank alongside antibiotics with their impact in the prevention of premature death. Until the early 1960s clinicians could only stand back and watch helplessly as their hypertensive patients inexorably deteriorated with heart failure, renal failure, coronary heart disease, strokes and dementia.

The dramatic reduction in stroke and coronary heart disease incidence over the last 10 years can, in part, be attributed to the advent of tolerable antihypertensive drugs. Furthermore, the 'whole patient' approach to the management of hypertensive patients has further contributed to the fall in heart attacks and stroke rates observed in most developed nations.

The purpose of this chapter is to review the results of the randomised trials of antihypertensive therapy, with particular reference to the large-scale and more reliable studies.

THE IMPORTANCE OF CLINICAL TRIALS

The current emphasis on the concept of evidence-based medicine means that no pharmacological preparation should be administered unless there is firm evidence from well-conducted, randomised, controlled trials that their use is beneficial. This is particularly important in hypertensive patients because the condition is usually symptomless; the decision to prescribe drugs on a long-term basis to otherwise fit people must be based on absolute proof that this is worthwhile. In addition, the fact that hypertension is so common means that the recommendation to give drugs to millions of people, with its cost implications, must be based on a large body of reliable data. The topic of hypertension has been particularly well served in this respect as a great many excellent clinical trials have been conducted. These initially concentrated on very severe hypertension but, as the years went by, trialists have turned their attention to milder

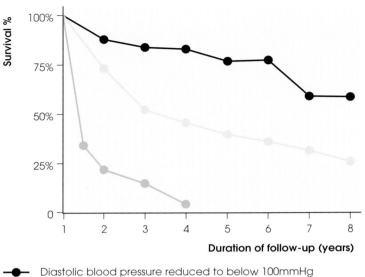

Figure 9.1
Survival rates for untreated and treated malignant hypertension.

—●— Diastolic blood pressure reduced to below 100mmHg

—●— Diastolic blood pressure remained above100mmHg

—●— Untreated malignant hypertension (*from Pickering 1968*)

cases where the immediate clinical risk of death is lower.

The pragmatic definition of hypertension is 'that level of blood pressure where investigation and treatment does more good than harm'. If this criterion is to be used then it is crucial that the clinician has an accurate knowledge of the usefulness of treatment, particularly of the milder grades of hypertension.

MALIGNANT HYPERTENSION

In this rare, but rapidly fatal condition, no formal trials were conducted because it was rightly felt to be ethically unjustifiable to withhold drugs that lowered blood pressure as soon as they became available. These were the ganglion-blocking drugs, hexamethonium and mecamylamine, which are no longer used because of their many side-effects. The clinical observation that with treatment these sick patients survived at all meant that drug therapy was mandatory. An 80% 2–year death rate was transformed to a 70–80% 5–year survival rate (Fig. 9.1).

RANDOMISED TRIALS OF HYPERTENSION TREATMENT

The introduction in the 1950s and 1960s of somewhat more tolerable drugs like methyldopa and the adrenergic neurone blockers (e.g. guanethidine) as well as the thiazide diuretics prompted the first wave of clinical trials, which concentrated on the more severe grades of hypertension where the risk of death was high. Subsequently, the introduction of the beta-blocking drugs in 1965 with their less marked side-effects led to the large numbers of trials of the treatment of mild hypertension.

Hamilton, Thompson and Wisniewski (1964)

This was the first randomised, controlled trial of drug therapy in relatively fit symptomless but severe hypertensive patients. Diastolic blood pressures exceeded 110 mmHg and, in more than half of the patients, the diastolic pressures were 130 mmHg or more. Ten men and 20 women received active drug therapy and 12 men and 19 women were treated with observation only. Amongst the men, eight vascular events (strokes and heart failure) developed in the untreated cases, whilst no events occurred in treated patients. In women there were eight events in those receiving no treatment and five in the treated group, a difference that was not statistically significant. However, in many of the treated women, blood pressures were not successfully reduced with the drugs available at the time. Hamilton and co-workers, therefore, re-analysed their data for women on the basis of whether or not diastolic blood pressure was reduced to below 110 mmHg. In 16 women, the blood pressure was successfully reduced and only one suffered a vascular event. In the 23 women whose blood pressures remained above 110 mmHg at follow-up, there were 12 vascular events. This was the only trial to provide information on the use of antihypertensive drug therapy in women until 1979.

Veterans administration (1967)

This was a placebo-controlled trial amongst patients similar to those studied by Hamilton and co-workers, but women were not included. Seventy men received active treatment whilst 73 received placebo, and entry diastolic pressures were between 115 and 129 mmHg. At follow-up, four deaths and 27 morbid events developed in the placebo patients compared with no deaths and two morbid events in the patients receiving active therapy.

Other trials of severe hypertension

Several other small-scale randomised trials were also conducted in the 1960s, but they provided little extra information when seen in isolation. In addition, there were some severe hypertensive patients included in the large-scale randomised trials discussed below, which had mainly concentrated on the milder grades of hypertension.

If the results of all of the trials of patients with diastolic pressures of 115 mmHg or more are pooled, then data are available on 1589 patients randomised to active therapy and 1629 control patients receiving no active treatment. Fatal or non-fatal strokes developed in 83 (5.2%) actively treated patients and 146 (9%) controls. Heart attacks developed in 109 (6.9%) actively treated patients and 147 (9%) controls.

By 1970, it was clearly established that it was no longer ethically justifiable to withhold drug therapy from patients with diastolic pressures of 110 mmHg or more. The trialists then turned their attention to the milder grades of hypertension where the individual patient's risk of death was less but, because of the large number of eligible people, the number of vascular complications was correspondingly greater.

Veterans administration (1970)

This trial was conducted in men with diastolic pressures between 90 and 114 mmHg. One hundred and ninety-four men received placebo tablets and 186 received active drugs. The results of this trial were impressive, with 35 morbid events and 16 deaths in the placebo group and nine morbid events and eight deaths in the active group. However, sub-group analysis of this study showed that the benefits were largely confined to patients with diastolic blood pressures between 105 and 114 mmHg. In the 170 men with entry diastolic pressures between 90 and 104 mmHg, 25% of placebo and 16% of actively treated patients suffered cardiovascular events, a trend that was not statistically significant. At this stage, it was generally considered that the reduction of coronary events with antihypertensive therapy was unimpressive, the benefits of antihypertensive therapy being largely related to prevention of strokes and heart failure.

The Hypertensive Detection and Follow-up Programme (HDFP 1979)

This is still a much criticised study, but its size means that reliable information can be obtained. Hypertensive patients were randomised either to 'stepped care' in specially established clinics or to 'referred care' with their usual health care facilities; 10 940 men and women were randomised and, at follow-up, more of the 'stepped-care' patients received active treatment than the 'referred-care' patients and average blood pressures were thus lower. In the strata of the HDFP study, which included mild hypertensive patients alone, there was an impressive reduction of both heart attacks and strokes, although it is difficult to be certain whether this effect was due to differences in blood pressure or to differences in quality of health care. One cynic commented that the HDFP was a randomised trial of socialised medicine with efficient delivery of health care rather than a trial of antihypertensive drug therapy.

Australian National Blood Pressure Study (ANBPS 1980)

This was a well-conducted, placebo-controlled trial of the use of chlorothiazide or placebo in 3427 men and women with diastolic blood pressures between 95 and 109 mmHg. At follow-up, 17 cerebrovascular events developed in the actively treated group and 31 events in the placebo group. These differences were statistically significant. The results for coronary heart disease were less impressive, with 98 cardiac events with active treatment and 109 events with placebo. There were 30 less deaths from all causes in patients who received diuretic treatment. The trial was terminated because of the significant reduction in strokes, leaving the question of coronary prevention unresolved.

The MRC trial of mild to moderate hypertension (1985)

The British MRC trial was also the source of much controversy. The entry diastolic pressures were between 90 and 109 mmHg and 17 354 men and women aged 35–64 years were randomised to placebo or active antihypertensive drugs. The actively treated group were further subdivided into half who received propranolol and half who received bendrofluazide in the astonishing dose of 5 mg twice daily. By the end of the study,

60 strokes occurred in the treated group and 109 in the placebo group, an effect that was statistically significant. No significant differences were found in overall rates of coronary events: 222 events occurred on active treatment and 234 in the placebo group.

The main problem with the MRC trial was that there were considerably fewer cardiovascular complications in the placebo group than was expected. This was due to the fact that the average diastolic pressure in these untreated patients fell to 90 mmHg or below soon after the trial started and remained at this level for 5 years. This is a problem with trials where the run-in period is inadequate. Blood pressures fall on rechecking and seem only to 'bottom-out' at the fourth visit. Another problem was the high drop-out rate from this trial, despite the fact that it was based in general practice.

The European Working Party on Hypertension in the Elderly (EWPHE 1985)

This well-conducted, randomised placebo-controlled trial was conducted in 840 men and women aged 60–99 years. Many of the findings are relevant to non-elderly patients, and the implications for the elderly are discussed in more detail in Chapter 15. By the end of the study, the 416 patients who received the diuretic-based regime suffered 48 heart attacks and 32 strokes. By contrast, in the placebo group, there were 59 heart attacks and 48 strokes. This trial was, therefore, the first to demonstrate convincingly coronary prevention as well as stroke prevention, and contrary to what some observers had expected, this was achieved with diuretic therapy. In this trial there was a significant reduction in cardiovascular deaths, a benefit that had eluded the previous trials. This was also the first trial to concentrate on the elderly, a hitherto neglected group despite their high absolute risk of cardiovascular death. The benefits of treatment were impressive.

The Coope and Warrender trial (1986)

In this general practice-based study of elderly patients aged 60–79 years in England and Wales, 419 men and women were randomised to receive the beta-blocker atenolol whilst 465 were given no active therapy. Atenolol alone proved ineffective in a great many patients, so a thiazide diuretic had to be added. As with other trials, there was a significant reduction in strokes, although in this study there was little impact on coronary heart disease despite the use of beta-blockers as first-line therapy.

The Systolic Hypertension in the Elderly Programme (SHEP 1991)

This was a multicentre trial in which 4736 patients aged 60 or more years were randomised to receive either chlorthalidone or placebo tablets. Of the participants, 42% were aged less than 70 years, so many of them were not particularly elderly. This trial broke new ground because it was conducted amongst patients with systolic pressures of more than 160 mmHg but diastolic pressures below 90 mmHg. Epidemiologists had long known that systolic blood pressure was a better predictor of cardiovascular risk than diastolic pressure but this was the first trial to investigate the value of reducing systolic pressures. At follow-up, there were only minor differences in diastolic pressures

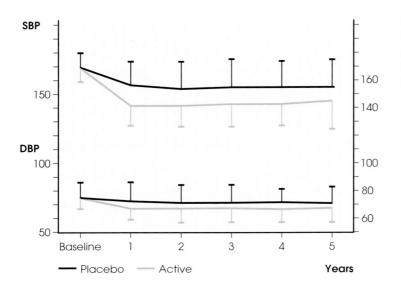

Figure 9.2
Baseline and follow–up blood pressure in the Systolic Hypertension in the Elderly Program (SHEP).

between treated and placebo patients, but the reduction in systolic pressures was significant (Fig. 9.2).

The results after 5 years were spectacular, with statistically significant reductions of both heart attacks and strokes and reduction in heart failure, TIA and the need for coronary revascularisation (Fig. 9.3). The trial included a highly selected group of patients and has its critics. However, in the light of this trial, it can now be said that the treatment of isolated systolic hypertension has been validated, although the level of systolic pressure at which treatment should be given remains uncertain.

The Swedish Trial of Old People with Hypertension (STOP-H 1991)

This multicentre trial of the treatment of diastolic hypertension largely confirmed the

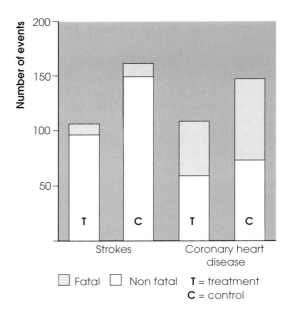

Figure 9.3
Results of treatment in the SHEP study.

findings of all other studies, with a significant reduction in strokes and some coronary prevention. It is not possible to be certain whether one drug group was better than another in coronary prevention.

The MRC trial of hypertension in the elderly (1992)

This second MRC trial was conducted in 4396 men and women aged 65–79 years who were randomised to receive either atenolol, a diuretic or placebo therapy. By the end of the study, there was a 25% reduction in strokes and a 19% reduction in coronary events in actively treated patients when compared with those receiving placebo tablets. Again, coronary prevention was achieved in the diuretic-treated patients but there was no prevention in patients randomised to the beta-blocker.

Some of the patients included for this trial were recruited on the basis of raised systolic blood pressures with diastolic pressures below 90 mmHg. A sub-group analysis of this group revealed that the treatment of isolated systolic hypertension led to a reduction in both heart attacks and strokes, a finding similar to that of the SHEP study.

The Shanghai Trial of Nifedipine in the Elderly (STONE 1996)

This trial is important because it was the first to investigate the value of blood pressure reduction with the newer hypertensive drugs. Hitherto, all the trials had only tested the thiazide diuretics or the beta-blocking drugs. The trial became more important also because of the anxieties about the safety of the calcium-channel blockers following the

publication of a series of retrospective case control studies in 1995. These suggested that the calcium-channel blockers might cause heart disease, cancer and gastrointestinal haemorrhage.

In the STONE study, 1632 patients aged 60–79 years with blood pressures greater than 160/95 mmHg were randomised to receive nifedipine or placebo. This trial, being conducted in a Chinese population, could provide no useful information on coronary heart disease as this condition is rare in China. There was, however, a statistically significant reduction in strokes (16 in the nifedipine group and 36 in the placebo group) and, importantly, no excess mortality from cancer or other non-cardiovascular diseases.

European trial of the treatment of isolated systolic hypertension in the elderly (SYST–EUR 1997)

This major international trial was published in 1997, and again the results were important in the light of the anxieties about the safety of the calcium-channel blockers. The study was conducted in men and women aged 60 years or more who had diastolic blood pressures below 95 mmHg and systolic blood pressures between 160 and 219 mmHg. Of these, 2398 patients were randomised to receive the short-acting channel blocker, nitrendipine, and 2297 patients received placebo tablets. The median follow-up period was 2 years. The SYST-EUR trial was terminated because of a highly significant reduction in strokes (42%). Myocardial infarction was reduced by 30%, although this trend was not statistically significant. However, there was a significant (25%) reduction of fatal and non-fatal cardiac endpoints, including sudden death (Fig. 9.4).

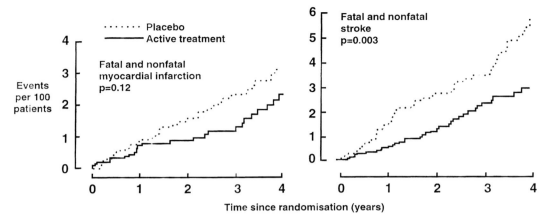

Figure 9.4

Syst-Eur Trial results.

The implications of the SYST-EUR trial are that the treatment of isolated systolic hypertension in the elderly is now fully vindicated and efforts should now be directed towards ensuring that this treatment is provided to the millions of eligible patients. The second important point is that this trial lays to rest any worries that the calcium-channel blockers might be harmful, as there were fewer cancers or episodes of haemorrhage in the patients randomised to receive nitrendipine compared with placebo. Finally, the SYST-EUR and STONE trial results mean that the guidelines on the treatment of hypertension published by the British Hypertension Society and other organisations will have to be re-written. Most guideline committees in the early 1990s had observed that only the beta-blocking drugs and the thiazide diuretics had been tested in outcome trials and shown to prevent the complications of hypertension. For this reason, these drugs were considered to be the preferred option.

This statement is no longer true as the calcium-channel blockers have now been shown to prevent heart attacks and strokes. In the SYST-EUR trial, about 40% of the patients receiving nitrendipine also received enalapril as add-on therapy, which strongly suggests that the ACE inhibitors can also be considered to be effective in the primary prevention of hypertension-related cardio-vascular disease.

THE BENEFITS OF TREATING MILD HYPERTENSION

A major overview or meta-analysis of many of the above studies, together with several other smaller studies that individually lacked the power to prove anything or showed only non-significant trends, was conducted in Oxford in 1994 (Fig 9.5).

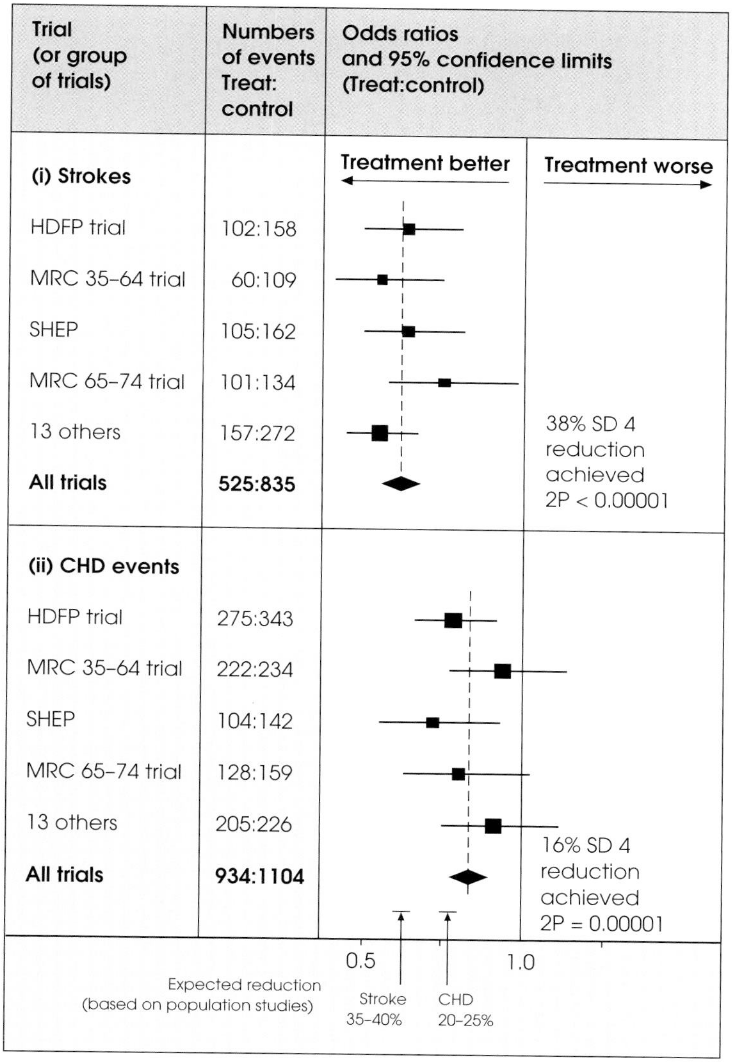

Trial (or group of trials)	Numbers of events Treat:control	Odds ratios and 95% confidence limits (Treat:control)	
		Treatment better	Treatment worse
(i) Strokes			
HDFP trial	102:158		
MRC 35–64 trial	60:109		
SHEP	105:162		
MRC 65–74 trial	101:134		
13 others	157:272		38% SD 4 reduction achieved 2P < 0.00001
All trials	**525:835**		
(ii) CHD events			
HDFP trial	275:343		
MRC 35–64 trial	222:234		
SHEP	104:142		
MRC 65–74 trial	128:159		
13 others	205:226		16% SD 4 reduction achieved 2P = 0.00001
All trials	**934:1104**		
Expected reduction (based on population studies)		0.5 1.0 Stroke CHD 35–40% 20–25%	

Figure 9.5
Meta–analysis of pooled results from the randomised trials of blood pressure reduction.

On the basis of epidemiological follow-up data from several large population surveys, the authors calculated that antihypertensive treatment for mild hypertension would be expected to bring about a 35–40% reduction in strokes and a 20–25% reduction in coronary heart disease events. Taking the results of all the outcome trials together, it was noted that the reduction in strokes was 38% while the reduction in coronary heart disease events was 16%.

Thus, the prevention of strokes was shown to be exactly on target and the prevention of coronary heart disease to be

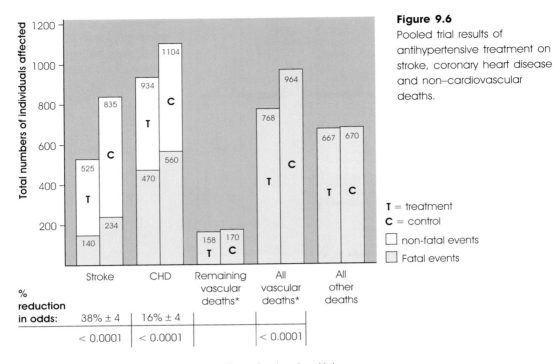

Figure 9.6
Pooled trial results of antihypertensive treatment on stroke, coronary heart disease and non-cardiovascular deaths.

T = treatment
C = control

☐ non-fatal events
☐ Fatal events

All available evidence from randomised antihypertensive drug trials (mean DBP difference 5 – 6 mmHg for 5 years)

* Includes any deaths from unknown causes

not significantly less than what would be expected. In general, the coronary prevention was less impressive in the younger patients, and it was this finding that led some earlier commentators to take the erroneous view that antihypertensive treatment was ineffective in coronary prevention.

There has been some speculation that the unimpressive effects on coronary prevention in the MRC trial of 35–64 year olds was due to the high dose of bendrofluazide used, with its adverse effects on plasma lipid and potassium levels. Later trials used lower doses of thiazides, which are equally effective at reducing blood pressure but have fewer biochemical effects. Another factor is that, over the age of about 65, epidemio-logical studies have demonstrated that plasma lipid levels may be less predictive of heart disease, so that the small rise in plasma cholesterol in older patients may be less important.

Antihypertensive therapy and death

The Oxford meta-analysis has the statistical power to demonstrate that antihypertensive treatment is capable of preventing both fatal and non-fatal strokes and heart attacks, with a statistically significant reduction of deaths from all vascular diseases, and no adverse impact on deaths from all other causes.

Antihypertensive treatment definitely saves lives and has no adverse effects on cancer or other illnesses (Fig. 9.6).

Clinicians can now be confident that their treatment is worthwhile in preventing strokes, heart attacks and premature deaths, with no adverse effects on other diseases.

Hypertension Optimal Treatment (HOT) trial

The final results of the HOT study were published in June 1998. The trial addressed two issues. Firstly, it attempted to answer the simple question 'How far should we lower the pressure?' The second objective was to investigate the value of low-dose (75 mg) aspirin in the treatment of mild hypertension. A total of 18 790 patients were randomised to one of three ranged diastolic pressures (below 80, 80–85 or 86–90 mmHg) and they received either placebo or active aspirin.

No significant differences in outcome were seen when comparing the three groups in relation to their target pressures. However, when the data from all three groups were pooled, the optimum effect on major cardiovascular events was seen in patients with diastolic pressures of 83 mmHg and systolic pressures of 138.5 mmHg (Fig. 9.7). This study does, therefore, allay any anxieties about a possible J-curve; there had previously been some anxieties that the reduction of diastolic pressures to below 80 mmHg might be harmful, particularly in patients with pre-existing heart disease. In the HOT study patients with heart disease at entry benefitted most if their diastolic pressures were reduced to below 80 mmHg, as did the sub-group with diabetes mellitus.

The patients randomised to receive aspirin had a 15% reduction in myocardial infarction. There was no impact on stroke

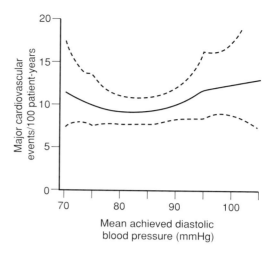

Figure 9.7

Incidence (95% CI) of major cardiovascular events in relation to achieved mean diastolic BP in the HOT study.

prevention and no excess of major haemorrhagic events.

Another important finding in the HOT trial was that lowering diastolic pressures to below 80 mmHg was not associated with any adverse effects on quality of life or major symptoms.

The HOT investigators commented that aspirin can be recommended 'provided the blood pressure is well controlled and the risk of gastrointestinal and nasal bleeding is carefully assessed'.

TRIALS STILL IN PROGRESS

Hypertension in the Very Elderly Trial (HYVET)

This trial is examining the possible value of treating hypertension in patients aged over

80 years. Some epidemiological studies of the very old suggest that the height of the blood pressure becomes a less powerful predictor of strokes or heart disease over the age of around 80 years, at least in the short term. However, the value of reducing high blood pressures over this age does need to be investigated. Benefits from blood pressure reduction were seen in patients over 80 years in the SHEP trial, but not in the EWPHE study.

Trials of new generation antihypertensive drugs versus the thiazides and the beta-blockers

Now that most of the trials designed to investigate whether blood pressure lowering is worthwhile have been completed, the next question is whether any one drug class is better than the others at preventing heart attacks and strokes. In particular, it is necessary to investigate whether the newer drugs (the calcium-channel blockers, the ACE inhibitors and the angiotensin-receptor antagonists) are as effective, or more, or possibly less effective than the long established beta-blockers and thiazides. It is interesting to note that the use of nitrendipine in the SYST-EUR trial was almost equally as effective at stroke prevention (42%) and more effective at preventing heart attacks (30%) than beta-blockers or thiazides in the meta-analysis in Fig 9.5. However, trials of 'new versus old' drugs are difficult to conduct as there is no placebo control group for comparison (that would no longer be ethical).

It is not likely that any results will be available until after the year 2000. However, the implications of these trials are important, not least in terms of the relative costs of the newer drugs.

In the meantime, trials in special groups have provided us with some information.

The ACE inhibitors have been shown to be effective in the secondary prevention of myocardial infarction in patients with left ventricular dysfunction, and these drugs have also been shown to delay the deterioration of renal function in both diabetics and non-diabetics with nephropathy. Furthermore, verapamil (but not nifedipine) has been shown to be effective in the secondary prevention of myocardial infarction both in normotensive and hypertensive patients. It is, however, uncertain whether it is possible to extrapolate from these trials conducted amongst highly selected patients to other patients with uncomplicated hypertension.

Swedish Trial of Old People with Hypertension (STOP-H-2)

This is an open labelled study in which patients are randomised to be prescribed a diuretic with or without a beta-blocker, or a calcium-channel blocker with or without an ACE inhibitor. This is being conducted amongst elderly patients.

Antihypertensive and Lipid-Lowering Heart Attack Trial (ALLHAT)

In this trial in the USA, patients are randomised to receive either a diuretic, an ACE inhibitor, a calcium-channel blocker or an alpha-blocker. In addition, where relevant, patients are also randomised to receive a lipid-lowering agent or a placebo.

Anglo–Scandinavian Cardiac Outcome Trial (ASCOT)

In this trial, patients are randomised to receive either atenolol, to which a thiazide is added if necessary, or amlodipine, to which enalapril is added if necessary. In addition, patients with modestly raised serum cholesterol levels are also randomised to receive the lipid-lowering drug atorvastatin or placebo. Patients with plasma cholesterol levels greater than 6.5 mmol/l are considered to require lipid-lowering drugs anyway and it was considered not ethical to do a placebo-controlled trial in this group. The ASCOT patients are required to be at high risk with at least three adverse cardiovascular risk factors. The first patients were entered into this study in 1998.

Losartan Intervention For End-point Trial (LIFE)

This is a trial established by a pharmaceutical company, which compares an angiotensin-receptor antagonist (losartan) with atenolol in hypertensive patients with left ventricular hypertrophy (LVH) on their ECG. These patients are therefore also at high risk. Recruitment for this trial was completed in May 1997 with 18 000 patients enrolled in Scandinavia, the UK and USA.

There are several other long-term studies in special high-risk groups, largely sponsored by the pharmaceutical companies. In particular, these studies are investigating the ACE inhibitors or the angiotensin-receptor antagonists in high-risk patients, including those who have recovered from a stroke or who have had a heart attack or have renal impairment. Details of the design of many of these trials have not yet been published.

WHO BENEFITS FROM ANTIHYPERTENSIVE THERAPY?

As stated earlier, all the national and international guidelines that were published in

1993 are now out of date since the publication of the STONE the SYST-EUR and the HOT trials and the advent of the angiotensin-receptor antagonists. New guidelines became available during 1997 and 1998 which recommended more aggressive control of blood pressure at all ages, and endorsed the use of more modern drugs in a larger proportion of patients.

Diastolic blood pressure

If the diastolic blood pressure consistently exceeds 90 mmHg then, up to the age of 80 years, antihypertensive drugs should be prescribed. The only exception to this rule is that the threshold can be raised to 95 mmHg in very low risk patients, mainly premenopausal women who are nonsmokers with below average serum cholesterol levels.

Systolic blood pressure

We suggest that at all ages antihypertensive drugs should be prescribed if the systolic blood pressure consistently exceeds 160 mmHg.

Target level of blood pressure

On the available evidence we are confident that systolic blood pressures should be reduced to below 140 mmHg and systolic blood pressure to below 85 mmHg.

A study from Glasgow has demonstrated that the outlook for a hypertensive patient is more closely related to the height of the blood pressure whilst on treatment rather than the initial severity of the hypertension (Fig 9.8). The findings in population surveys of poor control of blood pressure in the

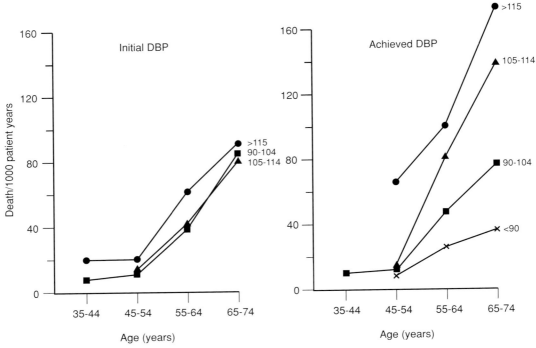

Figure 9.8
Age-specific mortality rates in 1162 men whose blood pressures were measured at entry to the clinic and thereafter during treatment. At all ages, the influence of achieved blood pressure on mortality was greater than that of initial blood pressure.

majority of hypertensive patients are therefore particularly alarming (see Chapter 2).

Complicated hypertension

The topic of hypertension in the presence of its vascular complications is covered in Chapter 14. In general, in these high-risk patients the threshold for instituting antihypertensive medication should also be 160/90 mmHg.

It is important to take into consideration the absolute cardiovascular risk status of individual patients, and clinicians should take an active role in controlling plasma lipid levels and, where relevant, persuade their patients to stop smoking.

How representative are patients in long-term clinical trials?

There is a tendency amongst some clinicians to extrapolate directly from the results of the trials discussed here and to draw attention to the fact that a great many patients (often thousands) had to receive antihypertensive drugs in order to prevent one heart attack or one stroke. We believe that this can be a very misleading statistic as it only takes into account the absolute benefits of treatment in the participants of these particular trials. Patients who agree to co-operate in these long-term studies are not representative of hypertensive patients in general. They tend to be rather well-to-do and have a low overall cardiovascular risk (with a low prevalence of cigarette smoking). Afro-Caribbean and Asian patients tend to be under-represented. Most participants have no evidence of end-organ damage at the outset, and few have LVH (a powerful risk factor).

As the absolute number of cardiovascular events is often low, many thousands of participants are required if significant results are to be obtained and the trials take many years. It is not, therefore, correct to extrapolate directly from these trial results to patients in more normal clinical practice, where LVH, proteinuria and other risk factors are likely to be more common. In this respect, the results of the much criticised HDFP study more readily reflect clinical practice as there were many high-risk patients and African Americans were included. It is better, therefore, to concentrate on the relative benefits of treatment in the trials (i.e. a 38% reduction of strokes and a 16% reduction in heart attacks) rather than the absolute benefits in the low-risk trial participants. These relative benefits appear to be roughly similar at all grades of blood pressure elevation, including very high risk, severe hypertensive patients.

CONCLUSIONS

Antihypertensive therapy is successful in preventing both heart attacks and strokes. The outcome for a hypertensive patient is more closely related to the accuracy of blood pressure control with therapy, rather than the height of the blood pressure at first presentation. Severe hypertensive patients with good blood pressure control do well, whereas milder cases with poor control do badly. The prime concern for clinicians and public health staff must be to ensure that this well-validated treatment is effectively provided for all who need it.

FURTHER READING

Alderman MH, Cushman WC, Hill MN, et al. International round table discussion of national guidelines for the detection, evaluation and treatment of hypertension. Am J Hypertens 1993; **6**: 974–81.

Collins R, MacMahon S. Blood pressure, antihypertensive drug treatment and the risks of stroke and of coronary heart disease. Br Med Bull 1994; **50**: 272–98.

Collins R, Peto R, MacMahon S, et al. Blood pressure, stroke and coronary heart disease. Part 2 short term reductions in blood pressure: overview of randomised drug trials in their epidemiological context. Lancet 1990; **335**: 827–38.

Hansson L et al for the HOT Study Group. Effects of intensive blood-pressure lowering and low-dose aspirin in patients with hypertension: principal results of the Hypertension Optimal Treatment (HOT) randomised. Lancet 1998; **351**: 1755–62.

Isles CG, Walker LM, Beevers DG, et al. Mortality in patients of the Glasgow Blood Pressure Clinic. J Hypertens 1986; **4**: 141–56.

Sever PS, Mackay JA. The hypertension trials. J Hypertens 1996; **14**(Suppl 2): S29–S34.

Staessen JA, Fagard R, Thijs L, et al for the Systolic Hypertension in Europe (Syst-Eur) Trial Investigators. Randomised double-blind companison of placebo and active treatment for older patients with systolic hypertension. Lancet 1997; **350**: 757–64.

Non-drug Control of Blood Pressure

Background

Studies in the general population in Western countries have shown that approximately 20% of adults have a raised blood pressure, with either a diastolic pressure greater than 90 mmHg or a systolic pressure greater than 160 mmHg on first measurement (see Chapter 1). In this group there is an increased risk of cardiovascular disease, which is related to the height of the blood pressure. Also at risk are those in the upper half of the normal distribution, i.e. around 50% of the population.

Many people found at screening to have blood pressure above the upper limits of normal for their age may normalise their pressure on re-measurement on a subsequent visit. However, in about 10% of the adult population, blood pressures remain above the threshold where drug treatment would be considered to be necessary. The prospect of so many people taking antihypertensive drugs must be viewed with alarm. Clearly, every effort needs to be focused on whether we can lower blood pressure without drugs when it is near to or above the upper range of normal, by means of lifestyle alterations. Furthermore, it is possible that these alterations, if applied on a population-wide basis, might help to prevent this development of hypertension in the first place.

Increasing evidence does suggest that various changes, particularly in the diet, may lower blood pressure and that these changes in lifestyle are additive to some antihypertensive drugs.

These changes in lifestyle should also be designed to reduce the other cardiovascular risk factors for premature vascular disease, namely tobacco consumption, high blood lipid levels and diabetes.

EFFECT OF OBSERVATION

Repeated measurement of blood pressure during follow-up usually causes a fall in blood pressure. This was best seen in the MRC trial of mild hypertension where a group of patients was treated either with propranolol, bendrofluazide or a placebo. In addition, one small group of patients were observed without any treatment but all had the same measurements of blood pressure. All patients were seen at regular intervals during the trial and there was a fall in blood pressure in all four groups. In those receiving either the beta-blocker or the diuretic this fall was only just significantly greater than in the changes in the untreated patients. Another finding was that placebo tablets had no additional effect on blood pressure compared with the group on follow-up alone with similar measurements of blood pressure. This fall in blood pressure reached a maximum at 3 months and there was no further fall with observation or placebo after this. This phenomenon is partly due to the trend for abnormal clinical indices to regress (or rise) towards the group average on rechecking. In the case of blood pressure there is also the effect of the patient's acclimatisation to the clinical environment and familiarisation with clinical measurement techniques.

The results of the MRC trial allow us to draw three important conclusions:

1. Patients with mild hypertension who have their blood pressure measured regularly will, as a group, sustain a fall in blood pressure. It is important, therefore, not to rush into treatment, either with non-drug or drug therapy.
2. If non-pharmacological therapy is started within the first 3-month period, the blood pressure fall may falsely be ascribed to the intervention when in fact it may only be due to the re-measurement of blood pressure alone.
3. These findings clearly indicate that it is essential in any blood pressure-lowering clinical trial, with non-drug or drug therapy, to have proper control groups to allow for the effects of clinical observation alone.

DIETARY ALTERATION

Increasing evidence suggests that the high incidence of cardiovascular disease in some Western countries compared with others is largely related to differences in diet, and particularly differences in sodium, potassium and saturated fat intake, combined with a relative lack of fruit and vegetables. There is now accumulating evidence that alteration of sodium and potassium intake, even in those who already have raised blood pressure, may cause substantial falls in blood pressure.

Alteration of salt intake

Historical perspective

Salt plays a vital role in regulating the amount of extracellular fluid. During evolution, as animals moved away from the sea, salt was in short supply, particularly for those herbivorous animals that were dependent on the very small amounts of salt present in plants. Animals adapted by developing very powerful mechanisms to conserve sodium. Humans, therefore, only need a salt intake estimated to be between 1 and 10 mmol/day (0.05–0.5 g salt).

About 4000 years ago, the Chinese discovered that salt had the 'magic' property of preserving food. This ability, particularly during the winter, was essential to the development of settled communities. Salt, therefore, became a valuable commodity and the main source of trade throughout the world. Much of the wealth of Venice in the 15th century was founded on the salt trade.

Once food is consumed that has been preserved in salt, the oral taste receptors become accustomed to the high salt concentration and natural foods taste bland. When salt became more readily available it was added to fresh food to bring it up to the same concentration as in preserved food.

With the invention of the deepfreeze and the refrigerator, food can now be preserved without the addition of salt. Nevertheless, we continue to add large amounts of salt unnecessarily to our food, so that salt intake in most Western countries is between 150 and 300 mmol/day (equivalent to 9–12 g salt/day). There is now very strong evidence in animals, and accumulating evidence in man, that this unnecessarily high salt intake is an important precipitating or underlying cause for the development of high blood pressure. Growing evidence now suggests that we should all reduce our salt intake in order to reduce the number of people that develop hypertension and to lower the whole population's average blood pressure. Indeed, in most countries expert committees have advised that this should be done. In the UK, for example, the COMA cardiovascular report recommended a population-wide reduction in salt intake of 30%, from 9 to 6 g/day. This is in line with similar recommendations in the USA.

Two French nephrologists, Ambard and Beaujard, in the early 1900s were the first to show that severe restriction of salt did lower blood pressure in patients with renal failure and hypertension. This work was largely ignored until Kempner in the mid-1940s found that a rice and fruit diet that was low in protein and sodium and rich in potassium was effective in patients with very severe hypertension. This diet, consisting of plain boiled rice and fruit, was widely used at the time, although patients found it difficult to tolerate. When the thiazide diuretics were introduced in the 1950s this severe form of salt restriction was abandoned and it was not until the early 1970s that more moderate forms of sodium restriction were first suggested to lower blood pressure.

Studies from all over the world have now demonstrated that a modest restriction of salt intake from 10 to 5 g/day does cause a fall in blood pressure, which is equivalent to the effect of a single drug, e.g. a beta-blocker or a thiazide diuretic. Studies have also shown that the greater the degree of salt restriction, the greater the fall in blood pressure (Fig. 10.1). Furthermore, several studies have shown that patients with more severe hypertension (Fig. 10.2), older patients and black patients respond better to salt restriction. This is because these patients have a less responsive renin–angiotensin system to salt restriction with a smaller rise in renin release and circulating angiotensin II levels. This inhibition of the normal compensatory response allows a larger fall in blood pressure. This also explains why the addition of drugs that block the renin system, such as the ACE inhibitors and the angiotensin-receptor antagonists, are particularly effective when combined with salt restriction.

A recent study in subjects over the age of 60 years has confirmed that a modest reduction in salt intake causes large reductions in blood pressure, equivalent to that seen with a thiazide diuretic, in both hypertensive and normotensive subjects. This indicates that older subjects should reduce their salt intake, a dietary change that is likely to have a major impact on the incidence of strokes in this high-risk group.

Our recommendation, therefore, is that all patients should reduce their salt intake. Some will find it easier to change their dietary habits if they eat at home and are able to avoid processed or convenience foods, which often have large amounts of added salt. After the initial 3–4 weeks when food tastes a little bland, particularly if large amounts of salt had been used previously, the taste receptors in the mouth become sensitive to lower concentrations of salt, so

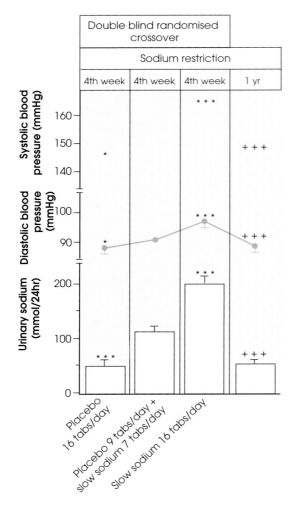

Figure 10.1
Effect of three salt intakes (10, 5 and 3 g/day) on blood pressure, showing a clear dose response, and 1-year follow-up where blood pressure remained controlled on 3 g salt intake.

patients find the same salt taste. If they return to the high-salt foods that they used to enjoy, these now taste unpleasant.

The assessment of salt intake

A dietary history is not an accurate way of assessing salt intake although it should still be undertaken. It is difficult to judge how much salt is in food in the first place, and how much that is added to cooking or at the table is actually consumed.

The best way to assess salt intake is to measure 24-hour urinary sodium excretion. More than 90% of sodium intake is excreted in the urine. However, sodium consumption varies from day to day depending on the food consumed, and urinary sodium excretion will follow these changes with an approximate 24-hour delay. One collection or, ideally, two consecutive 24-hour urine samples should give a reasonable estimate of whether a patient has a high sodium intake, i.e. more than 200 mmol sodium/day (equivalent to around 12 g salt/day), an average sodium intake around 150 mmol/day (approximately 9 g) or a reduced sodium intake of less than 80 mmol/day (approximately 5 g). Many patients are surprised by the amount of salt they consume when confronted with their 24-hour urinary sodium results. This is because salt is often hidden and high amounts may be present in processed foods. In people who live exclusively on processed food, 80–90% of the sodium intake may be in their food rather than added in cooking or at table.

How to reduce sodium intake

Any dietary change must be presented in an enthusiastic way and must fit in with the patient's lifestyle as well as the person who

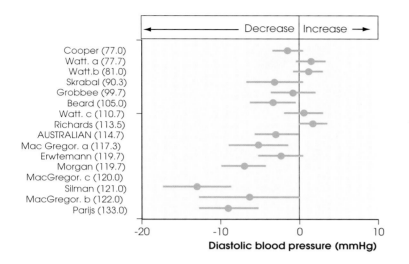

Figure 10.2

Effects of sodium restriction in different studies in order of severity of initial blood pressure. Figures in brackets represent the average mean arterial pressure on entry to the study.

does the cooking in the household. Changes in diet should be presented as a package, with a reduction in salt, an increase in potassium intake and a reduction in saturated fat with a lower cholesterol intake. Patients and, more importantly, whoever cooks in the household should be instructed as follows:

1. Never add salt to the food at the table.
2. Do not to add salt in the preparation of food and in cooking.
3. Avoid processed foods that have a high sodium content. This particularly applies to processed meat products, dried soups, ready prepared meals, take-away food and many restaurant meals.
4. Avoid flavour 'enhancers', e.g. stock cubes, gravy mixtures, soy sauce and monosodium glutamate.
5. Garlic, ginger, herbs, spices and chilli should be substituted for salt.

These simple steps can halve salt intake in patients, to around 80 mmol or 5 g/day. To reduce it further in most countries means finding a source of salt-free bread, as a slice of bread contains approximately 0.5 g salt. Where salt-free bread is available, it is possible to reduce salt intake to around 50 mmol or 3 g/day.

Many countries are introducing legislation that requires the salt content to be printed on the packaging of processed foods. However, patients may be confused by this as the salt content is expressed in grams of sodium per 100 g food.

One way to explain to patients how to judge the salt content of food is to compare it with sea water (Table 10.1). The salt content of cornflakes, some breads and processed foods is greater than sea water. By contrast, fresh food including fish and meat has a low salt content.

The optimum salt intake recommended by most experts is only one standard deviation below the population average. This means that many people are already consuming a

Table 10.1
Salt content of some common foods relative to seawater.

Processed foods	Sodium g/100 g food	Seawater equivalence (%)
Cornflakes	1.1	110
Bread	0.5–1.2	50–120
Cheese	0.6–1.4	60–140
Bacon	1.5–2.0	150–200
Sausage	0.9–1.2	90–120
Fresh foods		
Fresh meat	0.05	5
Fresh fish	0.05	5
Fresh vegetables	0.0–0.02	0–2
Fresh fruit	0.0–0.01	0–1

Note the difference between processed and fresh foods. Seawater contains 1.0 g sodium/100 g water. Therefore, it is easy to calculate when next in the supermarket the percentage seawater equivalence of processed foods. Most people find seawater somewhat unpleasant.

low-salt diet because they like good food, and this trend may be social class related. In the INTERSALT project, much of the difference in blood pressure between examinees in the highest and lowest social class was attributable to differences in salt intake.

The so-called 'salt controversy'

Until a few years ago there was controversy about the role of salt restriction in the treatment of high blood pressure, because of the poor quality of the trials. There is now no dispute that moderate salt restriction is an effective way of lowering high blood pressure. The pro-salt lobby, financed by the salt and food industry in the USA, UK and Europe, have continued to spend large amounts of money trying to confuse the issue. This is similar to the argument seen with cigarette smoking in the 1960s, where it was claimed that the evidence that smoking was harmful was not absolutely clear cut and more studies were needed before any action should be taken. This attitude is unhelpful, particularly to patients. More co-operation between the food industry and the medical profession could resolve this problem as it is quite unnecessary to add so much salt to processed food.

Increasing dietary potassium

There is good evidence that potassium has the opposite effect on blood pressure to sodium, and that a high potassium intake may slow down or prevent the development of high blood pressure both in animals and in man. In general, a high-salt diet is associated with a low potassium intake and a low-salt diet is associated with a high potassium intake in fruit and vegetables.

However, studies have shown that increasing potassium intake alone does have a blood pressure-lowering effect (Fig. 10.3). These studies mainly used potassium chloride, usually in the form of slow potassium (Slow K), as this made the studies more controlled and slow potassium placebo tablets could be used in double-blind studies. A meta-analysis of all these studies clearly demonstrated that increasing potassium chloride intake does cause a fall in blood pressure by an amount similar to that found with a beta-blocker or a thiazide diuretic used alone (Fig. 10.4). An important study from Italy demonstrated that dietary alteration of potassium, by eating more fruit and vegetables, has a similar effect on blood pressure. Potassium chloride tablets have no

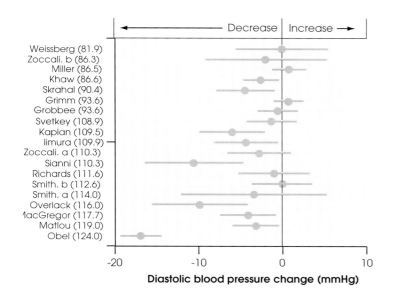

Figure 10.3
Effects of potassium supplementation in different studies in order of severity of initial blood pressure. Figures in brackets represent the average mean arterial pressure on entry to the study.

place in the non-pharmacological control of hypertension but a high potassium diet is useful and safe.

There is evidence in animals that increasing potassium and decreasing salt intake prevents strokes independently of blood pressure. Some epidemiological studies in man also suggest that a high potassium intake may protect from stroke, and a high-salt diet may increase the likelihood of stroke, an effect that again was independent of any effects on blood pressure.

How to increase potassium intake

Increasing potassium intake fits in well with the 'healthy diet'. Potassium is mainly present in fresh fruit and lightly cooked

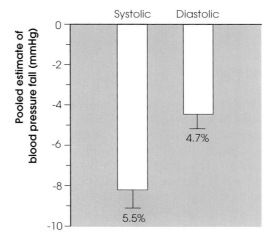

Figure 10.4
Pooled estimates of the treatment effect (and 95% CI) of potassium supplementation on blood pressure in untreated patients.

vegetables. It is also present, in high concentrations, in most fish. Increasing dietary potassium intake fits in with a reduction of salt and fat intake.

Salt substitutes

Salt substitutes containing potassium rather than sodium chloride have been used to help with compliance with salt restriction, and increase potassium intake. The major problem with pure potassium salt substitutes is that they taste unpleasant.

There are now several combinations of sodium and potassium chloride so-called 'salt alternatives' on the market. In general, these contain a smaller amount of salt (30–40%) and approximately 60–70% potassium chloride. In patients who feel that they must add some mineral to their food these may be useful. It is important to tell patients that other forms of salt (e.g. sea salt, rock salt and garlic salt) are identical to pure salt and should not be consumed.

Calcium

The role of a low calcium intake as a precipitating factor for high blood pressure remains uncertain. There was a suggestion that increasing calcium intake might lower blood pressure, but there is now evidence that increasing calcium intake in the diet has no significant blood pressure-lowering effect.

Magnesium

Magnesium, like potassium, is an important regulator of the excitability of cell membranes and is present in many foods. Magnesium sulphate is given intravenously in pre-eclamptic toxaemia to prevent convulsions and fits, but there is no secure evidence that it lowers blood pressure. In carefully controlled double-blind studies in patients with essential hypertension, disappointingly, magnesium supplements had no effect on blood pressure when compared with placebo. No specific recommendations for magnesium can be given to patients with high blood pressure at the present time.

Saturated fat and polyunsaturated fat

One study from Scandinavia reported that substituting saturated fat with polyunsaturated fat lowered blood pressure, but more recent trials have not confirmed this effect. Fish oil supplements have also been claimed to lower blood pressure but many studies have not been convincing. There is very strong evidence that high blood-cholesterol levels and high low-density lipoprotein (LDL) levels are important independent risk factors for arterial disease. Whilst cholesterol levels are in part due to the inherited differences in metabolism, they are also closely correlated with dietary saturated fat intake.

Raised plasma cholesterol levels greatly increase the risk of cardiovascular disease for a given level of blood pressure. A meta-analysis of the published trials of cholesterol lowering strongly suggests that reducing saturated fat intake, and thereby reducing cholesterol, does reduce the risk of cardiovascular disease. All hypertensive patients should have serum cholesterol levels measured and, whatever the level, they should be instructed to reduce their saturated fat intake. The degree of reduction of fat intake will obviously depend on the

Table 10.2

Simple dietary guide for patients with high blood pressure.

Reduced salt intake	do not add salt at table do not add salt to cooking avoid processed foods with high salt content (e.g. bacon, cheese, dried soups, etc – look at label)
Reduced saturated fat intake	reduce red meat and products (e.g. paté, sausages, etc) reduce milk products (fully skimmed milk allowed) reduce baked products with fat (e.g. pastries, biscuits)
Eat more	fish chicken and turkey fresh fruit and vegetables
Use	olive oil rape seed oil
Alcohol	maximum 21 units/week in men and 14 units/week in women

level of serum cholesterol and the ability of the patient to stick to the diet. Patients should be instructed to reduce or stop consumption of dairy products apart from fully skimmed milk, to avoid red meat and processed meat products and to consume more fresh fruit and vegetables, fish, particularly oily fish, and chicken. Where oil is essential, it is better to substitute a monosaturated fat such as olive oil or rape seed oil, but if this is not available the second best is a polyunsaturated fat such as sunflower or corn oil (Table 10.2).

The topic of hyperlipidaemia in hypertensive patients is covered in more detail in Chapter 14.

Dietary fibre

Dietary fibre consists of complicated carbohydrate substances that are not absorbed but decrease intestinal transit times and are useful in the prevention of constipation. One study suggested that increasing dietary fibre content might lower blood pressure. However, it was not clear whether this was a direct effect of the increase of fibre or due to concomitant alterations in sodium and potassium intake. Increasing fibre content in the diet has been claimed to prevent various intestinal diseases, particularly cancer of the colon, and may also have a cholesterol-lowering effect. Increasing fibre in the diet with a greater consumption of fruit and vegetables is worthwhile. However, many cereal products, which claim to be high in fibre, also have a high salt content.

Obesity and weight reduction

Many patients with high blood pressure are overweight, and there is no doubt from population studies that there is a close relationship between blood pressure levels and BMI, even when allowance is made for the tendency to overestimate blood pressure

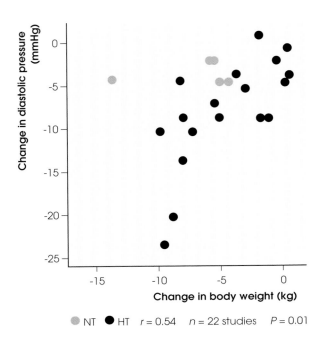

Figure 10.5

Fall in blood pressure related to reduction in weight. An overview of 22 studies.

in obese people. Well-controlled studies in patients with high blood pressure and obesity have shown that when they reduce their weight there is a fall in blood pressure. A 5 kg (11 lb) reduction in weight is associated with a 5 mmHg reduction in systolic pressure (Fig. 10.5). Some studies have reported that if the weight reduction is not associated with a reduction in salt intake the fall in blood pressure is smaller.

All patients, therefore, who are overweight and have high blood pressure should be encouraged to lose weight. In many patients with mild hypertension, weight reduction combined with salt restriction may bring blood pressure to a level where drug treatment is no longer indicated.

Alcohol

Epidemiological evidence strongly suggests that a high alcohol intake is associated with elevation of blood pressure and a fourfold increase in the risk of stroke. There is, however, some evidence that a moderate intake of alcohol, particularly in the form of red wine, may exert a modest protective effect against coronary heart disease.

The mechanisms of the alcohol–blood pressure link are uncertain and are almost certainly multifactorial. Acute alcohol consumption causes a rapid rise in blood pressure, presumably by a direct vasoconstrictor effect on some, but not all, vascular beds. Alcohol and its metabolites are sodium-transport inhibitors and this may provide some explanation of why vasoconstriction occurs.

Very heavy alcohol intake can cause severe hypertension by at least two mechanisms. Firstly, some alcoholic patients develop the alcoholic pseudo-Cushing's syndrome and blood pressure may be related to mineralocorticoid or glucocorticoid excess. Secondly, in heavy drinkers, the rise in blood pressure may be related to the stress of alcohol withdrawal rather than the effects of alcohol itself. In such patients, very high levels of plasma adrenaline and noradrenaline are found and a phaeochromocytoma-like crisis has been reported. Heavy drinkers, examined by the clinician the day after an evening with a high alcohol intake, may be in a state of subclinical alcohol withdrawal with resultant elevation of blood pressure. This state may not be immediately obvious to the clinician, who may mistakenly diagnose severe and pharmacologically resistant hypertension.

It is prudent to advise all people to avoid consuming more than the recommended maximum from the Expert Committees on Alcohol and Disease. The maximum weekly intake is 21 units (equivalent to 10.5 pints of beer or 4 bottles of wine) in men and 14 units in women (Table 10.3). It is also emphasised that binge drinking (which also causes strokes) should be avoided, and there should be one alcohol-free day in each week.

Many hypertensive patients consume more than the amounts suggested above, and with counselling are happy to moderate their intake whilst not going without the pleasures of social drinking. As described in Chapter 7, there are clinical and laboratory features that suggest that alcohol intake is too high. These are a plethoric appearance with central obesity, hyperuricaemia not due to diuretics or renal disease, a raised mean

Table 10.3
Maximum recommended alcohol intake.

	Men	Women
Units/week*	21	14
Beer (pints)	10½	7
Wine (glass)	21	14
Spirits (measures)	21	14
Sherry, etc (glass)	21	14

*1 unit of alcohol is equivalent to approximately 10 g.

corpuscular volume (MCV) and elevated levels of serum gamma glutamyl transferase. Otherwise, unexplained atrial fibrillation and inappropriate cardiomegaly suggest the diagnosis of alcoholic cardiomyopathy.

There are now many excellent randomised controlled trials that show that moderation of alcohol intake has a blood pressure-lowering effect, which is independent of any effect on caloric intake, or sodium and potassium (Fig. 10.6). This reduction can be achieved with sympathetic non-confrontational counselling, particularly by appropriately trained nurses in a primary health care setting.

SMOKING

Smoking is an independent risk factor for the premature development of arterial disease. Overwhelming evidence has demonstrated that stopping smoking is of benefit for the prevention of stroke, heart attack and peripheral vascular disease.

The mechanism whereby smoking may cause increased risk of arterial disease is not

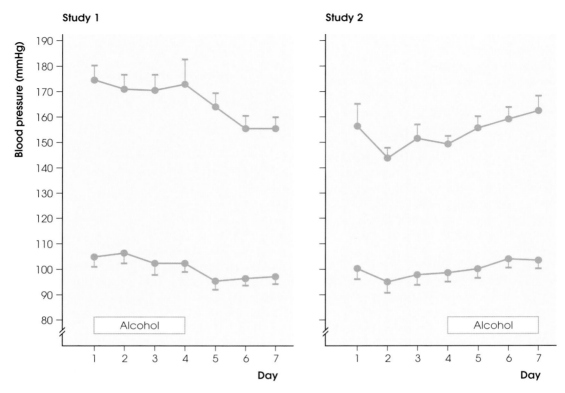

Figure 10.6
Change in blood pressure in hypertensive patients with cessation and restarting alcohol intake.

clear and may be related to a direct effect of nicotine or to the high levels of carbon monoxide in the blood that make the development of vascular disease more likely. Smoking is, after high blood pressure, the most preventable cause of death in the Western world. It is estimated that in the UK alone over 200 000 people per year die from smoking. Risks from smoking compound with the risks of high blood pressure and serum cholesterol levels.

However, whilst smoking a cigarette causes an acute rise in blood pressure, epidemiological evidence suggests that it has no effect on blood pressure in the long term. Indeed, blood pressure may be slightly lower in smokers compared with non-smokers, although malignant hypertension and renal artery stenosis due to atheroma are strongly associated with cigarette smoking. In view of the compounding risks of high blood pressure and smoking on premature vascular disease, it is particularly important that all patients with high blood pressure stop smoking. A careful explanation of the synergism between high blood pressure and smoking may produce a greater determination by the patient to give

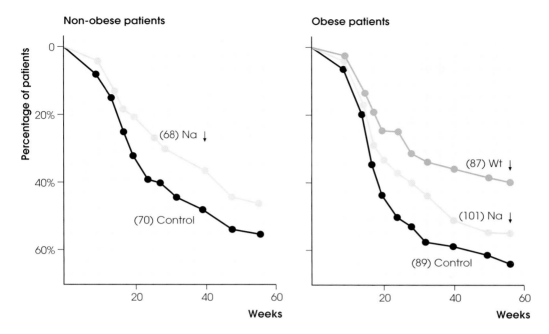

Figure 10.7
Proportion of hypertensive patients needing to restart drug therapy with no dietary advice (controls), weight restriction advice and salt restriction advice.

up. In middle-aged men, premature vascular disease, which, in part, will be brought on by cigarette smoking, may cause impotence, and this also may be a powerful motivating factor.

coffee intake does not seem to cause a fall in blood pressure.

COMBINED NUTRITIONAL ADVICE

CAFFEINE

Drinking a cup of coffee does cause an acute rise in blood pressure. However, epidemiological evidence does not show any relationship between caffeine consumption and blood pressure. Cutting back on

Several studies from the USA have demonstrated that when patients had their drug therapy withdrawn and were advised to restrict salt and alcohol intake and reduce weight, many did not need to restart their medication (Fig. 10.7). These studies, as well as the individual studies described in this chapter, strongly suggest that changes in diet in patients with hypertension should be presented as a package rather than on an individual nutrient level (Table 10.2). There is good evidence that the non-pharmacological dietary changes discussed in this chapter have a genuine synergistic effect with some antihypertensive drugs. This non-pharmacological advice should be given to all patients with raised blood pressure, irrespective of whether they are taking antihypertensive medication.

OTHER WAYS OF LOWERING BLOOD PRESSURE

Relaxation

The most effective way of lowering blood pressure is to sleep. This fall in blood pressure during sleep is largely due to relaxation of voluntary muscles. The reflex can be clearly demonstrated by relaxation of all muscles followed by the measurement of blood pressure. The thumb is then opposed against the index finger in isometric contraction and this will cause a marked increase in diastolic pressure of approximately 10–20 mmHg.

All relaxation therapies, for example biofeedback, transcendental meditation, yoga, sleep therapy and psychotherapy, use this simple, but basic, physiological reflex. One well-conducted randomised study did show a fall in blood pressure in both normotensive and hypertensive patients after relaxation therapy. However, more recent studies have demonstrated that this fall in blood pressure is due to patients learning to relax during the measurement of blood pressure in the clinic. The 24-hour ambulatory blood pressure profile was unchanged. It is sensible with all patients to review their lifestyle and ensure that they are not subjecting themselves to unnecessary stress, but there is little point in forcing those people who do not want to to relax.

Exercise

During dynamic exercise such as running, swimming or cycling, systolic pressure rises and diastolic pressure falls. In physically fit people, the rise in systolic pressure and heart rate are less. During isometric exercise, there is contraction of muscles without movement, and very large rises in both systolic and diastolic pressure.

Several studies have now demonstrated that regular exercise does cause a fall in blood pressure (Fig. 10.8). There is some debate about the amount of exercise needed, with different studies showing falls in blood

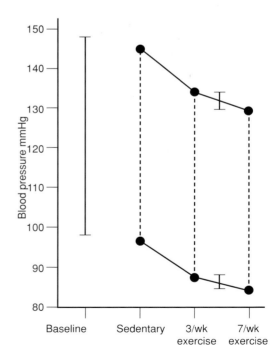

Figure 10.8

Effects on blood pressure of an exercise program, three or seven times a week.

pressure with widely differing amounts of exercise. Currently, our view is that, where appropriate, regular exercise should be done three to four times a week and the exercise should be sufficient to cause sweating. Patients who become fit often feel better, and this is sufficient reason in itself for encouraging patients to take exercise. However, sudden severe strenuous exercise may be harmful, particularly in patients who have coronary artery disease. Patients who are unfit should build up the exercise load slowly. Isometric exercise may be particularly harmful in patients with ischaemic heart disease.

FURTHER READING

Appel LJ, Moore TJ, Obarzanek E, *et al*. A clinical trial of the effects of dietary patterns on blood pressure. *N Engl J Med* 1997; **336**: 1117–24.

Cutler JA. Combinations of lifestyle modifications and drug treatment in management of mild–moderate hypertension: a review of randomized clinical trials. *Clin Exp Hypertens* 1993; **15**: 1193–204.

MacGregor GA, Markandu ND, Sagnella GA, *et al*. Double-blind study of three sodium intakes and long-term effects of sodium restriction in essential hypertension. *Lancet* 1989; **ii**: 1244–7.

Maheswaran R, Beevers DG. Effectiveness of advice to reduce alcohol consumption in hypertensive patients. *Hypertension* 1992; **19**: 78–84.

MRC Working Party on Mild to Moderate Hypertension. Randomised controlled trial of treatment for mild hypertension: design and pilot trial. *Br Med J* 1977; **2**: 1437–40.

Nelson L, Jennings GL, Esler MD, *et al*. Effects of changing levels of physical activity on blood pressure and haemodynamics in essential hypertension. *Lancet* 1986; **2**: 473–6.

Stamler R, Stamler J, Grimm R, *et al*. Nutritional therapy for high blood pressure. Final report of a four-year randomized controlled trial—the hypertension control program. *J Am Med Assoc* 1987; **257**: 1484–91.

World Hypertension League. Nonpharmacological interventions as an adjunct to the pharmacological treatment of hypertension: a statement by WHL. *J Hum Hypertens* 1993; **7**: 159–64.

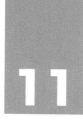

A Review of Antihypertensive Drugs

Background

Antihypertensive drugs were first introduced in the 1950s but, because of their side-effects, they were reserved for use in patients with very severe or malignant hypertension. Before their introduction, attempts to reduce blood pressure were made using either sedatives or tranquillisers like phenobarbitone, together with a very low salt diet. Some patients were even subjected to thoracolumbar sympathectomy or bilateral adrenalectomy. The first antihypertensive drugs were the ganglion-blocking drugs, such as hexamethonium, mecamylamine, pempidine and pentolinium. It soon became apparent that in patients with very severe hypertension, lives were being saved.

The subsequent introduction of the thiazide diuretics, methyldopa and adrenergic neurone blockers such as guanethidine, bethanidine and debrisoquine in the late 1950s and early 1960s meant that more tolerable blood pressure-lowering agents could be used in less severe hypertensives patients. Early clinical trials in 1964 and in 1970, where diuretics, reserpine and hydralazine were used, confirmed that these agents were also saving lives. However, all these agents, apart from the diuretics, had severe side-effects and are now obsolete.

In the mid-1960s the beta-blocker propranolol was introduced for the treatment of angina, and shortly afterwards it was found to lower blood pressure. The beta-blockers and the thiazide diuretics then became the mainstay of treatment for blood pressure in the 1970s and were employed in the randomised trials of the benefits of the treatment of mild to moderate hypertension. These trials (Chapter 9) clearly demonstrated a major reduction in stroke and coronary heart disease. Nevertheless, the beta-blockers and diuretics do have side-effects and in any case do not always control blood pressure. The search for newer drugs that are as effective at lowering blood pressure, and preventing heart attacks and strokes, but with fewer side-effects, has continued.

In the early 1980s, two new classes of compounds, the calcium-channel blockers and the ACE inhibitors, were introduced. These newer compounds are very effective at lowering blood pressure and have fewer or differing side-effects, with the potential advantage of fewer metabolic side-effects.

More recently, the angiotensin-receptor antagonists have emerged as a group of drugs with almost no side-effects and are now widely used. The outcome trials of the 'newer versus the old' antihypertensive drugs are discussed in Chapter 9.

WHICH DRUG FOR WHICH PATIENTS?

With the six main classes of drug available, the clinician and, more importantly, the patient has a wide choice of treatment options. Ideally, each patient should undergo some sort of assessment to decide which drug is the best tolerated and most effective in their particular case. After all, they are likely to need this treatment for the rest of their lives. Many of the newer drugs, whilst not having the serious side-effects of the older agents, may have more subtle effects and may reduce the quality of life on a long-term basis. A combination of a low dose of two different drugs with an additive effect may have fewer side-effects than higher doses of any one agent.

If one particular drug is not sufficiently effective, it is usually better to change to a different class of drug or to add a second agent in. These strategies are preferable to increasing the dose of the first agent. Schemes for reducing blood pressure are discussed in the next chapter. This chapter discusses the many drugs that are available, their mechanisms and their side-effects.

DIURETICS

Thiazide diuretics have been the backbone of blood pressure-lowering therapy since they were introduced in the 1960s. At that time they largely replaced rigorous salt restriction. More recently, there has been concern about their potentially harmful metabolic effects and the possibility that they may also cause arrhythmias in some patients. In men, impotence has emerged as a major problem with higher doses of the thiazide diuretics. In spite of these concerns, all the trial evidence suggests that diuretics do reduce strokes and also, particularly in the elderly, coronary heart disease. Clinical trial evidence suggests that in this regard they are more effective than the beta-blockers.

Diuretics are additive to nearly all antihypertensive drugs, particularly beta-blockers and ACE inhibitors. Before the advent of the calcium-channel blockers and ACE inhibitors, arteriolar vasodilators like hydralazine and minoxidil were often added to beta-blockers in resistant hypertension. However, these drugs caused sodium and water retention, offsetting the blood pressure-lowering effect. In this situation, powerful diuretics like frusemide had to be added in.

Thiazide diuretics

All thiazide diuretics have a fairly flat dose–response curve, so that increasing the dose has little further effect on blood pressure but markedly increases the metabolic consequences, e.g. lowered serum potassium, increased blood sugar and/or glucose intolerance, increased cholesterol and uric acid levels. Therefore it is best to use the minimum dose and nothing is gained by a dose increase.

There are only slight differences in the duration of action of the thiazides but major differences in dosage (Table 11.1). All are given once daily as their effect on blood pressure lasts for several days. Related sulphonamide compounds, such as chlorthalidone and metolazone, are longer acting and more powerful.

Mode of action

Thiazide diuretics act on the renal tubules to block sodium and chloride reabsorption. After a certain amount of sodium and water loss, compensatory mechanisms block these effects on the kidney so, within a few days, no additional loss of sodium occurs and total body sodium is maintained at a slightly reduced level. This causes a fall in the extra-cellular fluid volume and a small decrease in plasma and blood volume. With the loss of sodium and water, the kidney responds by increasing renin release, leading to the formation of the powerful vasoconstrictor angiotensin II. Therefore, the fall in blood pressure with a diuretic is largely determined by the fall in extracellular volume compensated by a reactive rise in plasma angiotensin II. This explains why diuretics are more effective in black patients and in older patients, who tend to have lower plasma renin levels and a smaller rise in renin and angiotensin II in response to volume depletion.

Beta-blockers partially inhibit the renin release caused by diuretics, and ACE inhibitors reduce the compensatory rise in plasma angiotensin II levels. For this reason, beta-blockers and ACE inhibitors are very effective when used in combination with a diuretic.

Table 11.1
Dosage of diuretics.

	Normal daily dose for hypertension
Thiazides	
Bendrofluazide	1.25–2.5 mg o.d.
Cyclopenthiazide	0.25 mg o.d.
Hydrochlorothiazide	12.5–25 mg o.d.
Thiazide related compounds	
Chlorthalidone	12.5–25 mg o.d.
Indapamide	1.25–2.5 mg o.d.
Metolazone	5 mg o.d.
Loop diuretics	
Bumetanide	1 mg b.d.
Frusemide	20–40 mg b.d.
Potassium sparing diuretics	
Amiloride	5–10 mg o.d.
Spironolactone	25–100 mg o.d.
Triamterene	50 mg o.d.

There is also evidence that thiazide diuretics have some direct vasodilating properties, which contribute to their antihypertensive effects. This may explain why the thiazides are more potent blood pressure-lowering drugs than the loop diuretics, despite the fact they are weaker diuretics.

Side-effects

Thiazides at low doses are reasonably well tolerated. They cause rare severe reactions, including rashes, thrombocytopenia and leucopenia. However, the MRC Mild Hypertension Trial showed that bendrofluazide causes impotence in many male patients (Fig. 11.1). Thiazides are therefore best avoided in sexually active men.

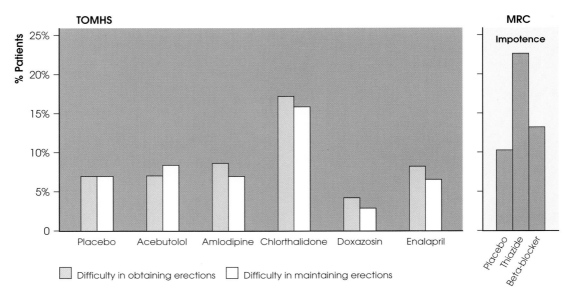

Figure 11.1
Thiazides and sexual function in men. Data from the Treatment of Mild Hypertension Study (TOMHS) and the MRC trial of mild hypertension.

Metabolic problems of thiazide diuretics

Hypokalaemia

Almost all patients treated with thiazides sustain a small fall in plasma potassium levels. This fall varies with the dose of the thiazide but varies from 0.3 to 1.0 mmol/l. Patients on a high salt intake will sustain a greater fall in plasma potassium with a diuretic, whereas in patients on a low-salt diet the fall in potassium is smaller. Whilst the dangers of hypokalaemia in patients with high blood pressure have not been clearly defined, circumstantial evidence suggests that it may be responsible for a high frequency of arrhythmias and sudden death. In the MRC Mild Hypertension Trial, there were more multifocal ventricular ectopic beats in thiazide-treated patients compared with those receiving either a beta-blocker or placebo. This effect may be increased by exercise. There is also evidence that patients who have suffered a heart attack have a worse prognosis if they have low plasma potassium at presentation.

Plasma potassium levels should be measured in all patients before starting diuretic therapy. If they are already low, further investigation is necessary to exclude primary or secondary aldosteronism. All patients who have started on diuretics should have a repeat plasma potassium check within a month or so of the start of treatment. In general, clinicians have neglected to watch plasma potassium levels, partly because mild hypokalaemia does not cause any obvious clinical effects.

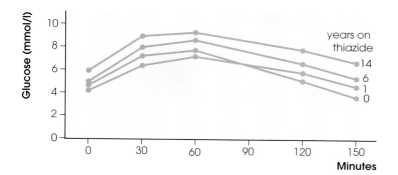

Figure 11.2
The long–term effect of thiazide diuretics on glucose tolerance.

How to avoid hypokalaemia on diuretics

Traditionally, potassium supplements were given. However, these also have side-effects, are not always effective and, in our view, are only rarely indicated. The amount of potassium in the combined thiazide and potassium formulations is trivial. The best way of minimising the fall in plasma potassium is to use low doses, e.g. 1.25 mg bendrofluazide or 12.5 mg hydrochlorothiazide. If thiazides are combined with ACE inhibitors or beta-blockers hypokalaemia is very uncommon as these agents suppress aldosterone release. Restricting salt intake will also reduce the fall in plasma potassium with the thiazide diuretics.

Thiazides are sometimes used with potassium-sparing diuretics like triamterene or amiloride. Whilst this may prevent hypokalaemia, it may occasionally cause more side-effects. Many of these combined preparations contain too much thiazide, and profound hypokalaemia and hyponatraemia has been described, particularly with moduretic, a combination tablet containing amiloride and hydrochlorothiazide.

If plasma potassium does fall to low levels with a low-dose thiazide diuretic it is likely that the patient has some other cause and a diagnosis of underlying primary aldosteronism should be considered.

Hyperuricaemia

All thiazide diuretics cause an increase in plasma uric acid levels and may occasionally precipitate gout. This effect is minimised if low doses are used. It is uncertain whether the symptomless rise in plasma uric acid levels has any long-term consequences. Hyperuricaemia is common in hypertensive patients, even without thiazides, but it is doubtful whether serum uric acid is an independent cardiovascular risk factor. Renal impairment and a high alcohol intake also cause an increase in serum uric acid.

Glucose intolerance

Hypertensive patients tend to have a degree of insulin resistance, and thiazide diuretics, given long term, may cause a further deterioration in glucose tolerance (Fig. 11.2). Some patients develop elevated blood glucose levels and, rarely, frank diabetes may be precipitated. In patients who already have diabetes mellitus there may be a slight worsening of diabetic control, and in patients receiving insulin the dosage may need to be increased slightly.

Patients with non-insulin dependent diabetes (NIDDM), controlled either by oral antidiabetic drugs or diet, should not be given thiazide diuretics unless absolutely necessary. Some patients may normalise their blood glucose levels by changing from a thiazide diuretic to another antihypertensive agent.

Blood lipids

Thiazide diuretics cause a small rise in plasma cholesterol and triglyceride levels with long-term treatment. This is mainly due to a rise in LDL cholesterol and, in some studies, a fall in HDL cholesterol. In theory, this might hasten the development of vascular disease and could partly offset the benefits of the reduction in blood pressure. However, the recent studies in the elderly that have used a thiazide diuretic regime have clearly demonstrated not only a reduction in strokes, but also in coronary heart disease.

Calcium

Thiazide diuretics can elevate plasma calcium levels into the range where a diagnosis of primary hyperparathyroidism should be considered. These drugs also reduce urinary calcium excretion and lead to a positive calcium balance. Several studies have demonstrated that in the long term they cause an increase in bone mass, and a reduction of hip fractures. This may be beneficial in postmenopausal women with high blood pressure.

Other problems

In patients who are sodium and water depleted, diuretics may cause further volume depletion. Patients with chronic renal disease may show a deterioration in renal function. Rarely, thiazides cause large falls in plasma sodium with frank hyponatraemia (e.g. serum sodium 110–125 mmol/l). Hyponatraemia may cause confusion, dehydration, vomiting and muscle weakness, particularly in the elderly.

A small rise in packed cell volume and haemoglobin level is common with diuretics. Both are potential risk factors for strokes. Thiazides also increase platelet aggregation, which might cause an increased tendency to develop thrombotic disease.

Thiazides should not be used for hypertension in pregnancy as they may reduce utero-placental blood flow (see Chapter 16).

Loop diuretics

The two most commonly used drugs in this class are frusemide and bumetanide. They act on the ascending limb of the loop of Henle and block sodium reabsorption. They are faster acting than the thiazides, and have the disadvantage of a shorter duration of action. They cause a loss of sodium and water within 2 to 3 hours, but during the rest of the day there is sodium and water retention. They are therefore not widely used in the treatment of hypertension. However, in patients with resistant hypertension they are used with other drugs, particularly the ACE inhibitors, and given twice daily so that they have a sustained effect on sodium balance. The loop diuretics have fewer metabolic side-effects than the thiazides. However, their rapid diuretic effect may cause great inconvenience to the patient.

Potassium-sparing diuretics

These drugs act on the distal renal tubule and reduce potassium excretion whilst increasing sodium and water loss. Currently there are three potassium-sparing diuretics available: spironolactone, triamterene and amiloride.

Spironolactone

Spironolactone is an aldosterone antagonist, which may also have a direct effect on the distal renal tubule. Given alone, usually in large doses, it can control blood pressure in patients with primary aldosteronism prior to surgery or in patients where surgery is contraindicated. It is also used in patients with non-tumourous aldosterone excess. However, spironolactone has endocrine side-effects, including gynaecomastia, loss of libido in men and intermenstrual or postmenopausal bleeding. It can also have gastrointestinal side-effects, particularly dyspepsia. In view of these side-effects, spironolactone is no longer recommended for the treatment of hypertension except in patients with primary aldosteronism.

Triamterene

This drug is less effective in lowering blood pressure than spironolactone, but it does partially block the potassium-lowering effect of thiazide diuretics. It has therefore been combined with thiazide diuretics to prevent the fall in plasma potassium.

Amiloride

Although structurally different to triamterene, amiloride has a similar action on the distal tubule. It has been widely marketed in combination with a thiazide diuretic, although the most widely used formulation contains 50 mg hydrochlorothiazide, which is excessive. Hyponatraemia and hypokalaemia may be provoked. There is now a half-strength dose containing 25 mg hydrochlorothiazide and 2.5 mg amiloride, although even this dose is too high. If a lower dose of thiazide is given, e.g. hydrochlorothiazide 12.5 mg, it is usually not necessary to add amiloride. However, amiloride is relatively free of side-effects and is a reasonable alternative for the treatment of primary aldosteronism, where spironolactone cannot be used.

All distal-acting diuretics may cause dangerous hyperkalaemia in patients with renal failure, so care must be taken in patients with any renal disease. Potassium-sparing agents may also cause hyperkalaemia when used with ACE inhibitors and this combination is not recommended.

Indapamide

This diuretic may be different from the thiazides, with additional blood pressure-lowering effects independent of the loss of sodium. It is uncertain whether it is more potent than the thiazides. It may have less adverse effects on glucose tolerance and has been promoted as being useful in patients with diabetes mellitus.

BETA-BLOCKERS

The beta-adrenergic receptor blockers were originally introduced in the early 1960s for the treatment of angina pectoris, and their blood pressure-lowering effects were not initially appreciated. During the 1970s and 1980s they became the mainstay of blood pressure-lowering treatment but, in view of their subtle side-effects, they have become less popular. They have been shown to reduce the risk of reinfarction in patients who have had a heart attack. However, in two randomised controlled trials, beta-blockers had no effect in preventing first myocardial infarctions and a smaller effect on stroke than the thiazide diuretics.

Mode of action

The beta-blockers compete with the endogenous catecholamines for adrenergic beta receptors. Beta receptors can be divided into two classes: $\beta1$ and $\beta2$ receptors. Blocking the $\beta1$ receptors reduces the heart rate and the contractility of the heart, with a concomitant reduction in cardiac output. This may be part of the mechanism of the blood pressure-lowering effect. Blockade of the $\beta2$ receptors causes vasodilatation in voluntary muscle but may cause bronchoconstriction, particularly in asthmatic subjects. Beta-blockers also inhibit renin release, leading to falls in plasma angiotensin II levels, which probably explains most of their blood pressure-lowering action. This also explains why beta-blockers are less effective in patients with low plasma renin levels, such as Afro-Caribbeans and older hypertensive patients.

Differences between beta-blockers

For all practical purposes, all beta-blockers are as effective as each other in reducing blood pressure. However, some differences between them have emerged.

Cardioselectivity

The cardioselective beta-blockers such as acebutolol, atenolol and metoprolol have a greater effect on cardiac $\beta1$ receptors. Some beta-blockers are not cardioselective (for example, propranolol and oxprenolol) as they block both $\beta1$ and $\beta2$ receptors. There does not appear to be any difference in the blood pressure-lowering effect between selective and nonselective beta-blockers.

Intrinsic sympathomimetic activity

Like many competitive inhibitors, some beta-blockers stimulate the beta receptors as well as block them, particularly when endogenous levels of catecholamines are low. This intrinsic sympathomimetic activity (ISA) or partial agonist activity is seen with pindolol, oxprenolol and, to a lesser extent, acebutolol. These agents are therefore less prone to cause bradycardia, but may possibly be less effective in lowering blood pressure.

Lipophilicity

Some beta-blockers are more lipid-soluble than others. Lipid-soluble (lipophilic) drugs are more likely to enter the brain and cause tiredness, sleep disturbance and vivid dreams. The less lipid-soluble, or hydrophilic, drugs such as atenolol, acebutolol and sotalol should cause less central side-effects. Lipid-soluble drugs are mainly metabolised by the liver, whereas water-soluble ones are excreted by the kidney. This is important if there is either hepatic or renal impairment and may influence the choice of beta-blocker.

Table 11.2

Daily dosage of beta-adrenoceptor blockers.

Acebutolol	200–800 mg
Atenolol	25–100 mg
Bisoprolol	5–10 mg
Metoprolol	50–400 mg
Nonselective beta-blockers	
Propranolol	80–360 mg
Beta-blockers with partial agonist activity	
Celiprolol	200–400 mg
Oxprenolol	80–320 mg

Table 11.3

The side-effects of beta-blockers.

Sleep disturbance	Heart failure
Nightmares	Reduction of exercise tolerance
Lethargy	Raynaud's syndrome
Bronchospasm	Claudication
Bradycardia	Impotence

Duration of action

Most beta-blockers reduce blood pressure within 1–2 hours of a single oral dose, and most of them can be given once daily. However, oxprenolol, propranolol and metoprolol are relatively shorter acting and are normally prescribed twice daily. By contrast, atenolol and bisoprolol are longer acting. In many patients, low doses of beta-blockers should be given, often with a reduction in side-effects. However, at lower doses the drugs may need to be given more often. Atenolol 12.5 mg (half tablet) once a day does not cover 24 hours, whereas the same dose twice a day may be effective (Table 11.2).

Side-effects of beta-blockers (Table 11.3)

Heart failure

When beta-blockers were first introduced, there was concern that they might precipitate heart failure, particularly in patients with damaged heart muscle. In patients with high blood pressure, where the left ventricle is performing well, beta-blockers are unlikely to precipitate heart failure. Patients with heart failure should not be given beta-blockers except under very carefully supervised conditions (see Chapter 14). In view of the slowing of AV conduction that beta-blockers can cause, they should not be given to patients with any form of heart block.

Reduction in peripheral blood flow

Because of the reduction in cardiac output and the reflex increase in peripheral resistance, all beta-blockers tend to reduce peripheral blood flow and cause cold hands and feet, particularly in colder climates. If symptoms are mild, advice about keeping hands warm and wearing gloves may suffice. However, they also worsen symptoms of Raynaud's disease and intermittent claudication. In severe peripheral vascular disease, gangrene has been precipitated by the use of beta-blockers. It is possible that beta-blockers with partial agonist activity, for example pindolol and oxprenolol, are less likely to do this. However, beta-blockers are best avoided and calcium-channel blockers or ACE inhibitors should be used instead.

Bronchospasm

All beta-blockers may precipitate bronchospasm, especially if there is a preceding history of asthma. However, an upper respiratory tract infection may precipitate asthma de novo in patients on a beta-blocker. It is claimed that the more cardioselective beta-blockers, such as atenolol, metoprolol, acebutolol and celiprolol, are less likely to have this effect. However, in our view, beta-blockers should not be given to anyone with asthma or who is likely to develop asthma.

Reduction in exercise tolerance

All beta-blockers cause a reduction in exercise tolerance, which can be a major problem for active young patients. Patients may feel tired when climbing stairs, particularly with a feeling of heaviness in the legs.

Central nervous system side-effects

Beta-blockers may cause sleep disturbance, vivid dreams and nightmares. These may be more common with the lipid-soluble beta-blockers such as propranolol and oxprenolol.

'Subtle' side-effects

Beta-blockers commonly cause a loss of drive and energy. These side-effects can be very subtle and are not always noticed by the patient but may be obvious to their spouse or other people. In the past the subtle effects of beta-blockers were ignored, but they are now the most common reason for not using or discontinuing therapy and

many clinicians now question the continued use of beta-blockers as first-line therapy.

Diabetes mellitus

Theoretically, beta-blockers can interfere with insulin secretion, but this a fairly minor effect. However, they can interfere with the metabolic response to hypoglycaemia in insulin-dependent diabetics, who also may not show the usual symptoms when they have become hypoglycaemic. This problem has been exaggerated however and, provided patients are advised appropriately, beta-blockers can be used in insulin-dependent diabetics, although ACE inhibitors are now the preferred first-line drugs in patients with diabetes (Chapter 14).

CALCIUM-CHANNEL BLOCKERS

Also known as the calcium entry antagonists, the CCBs were known to lower blood pressure many years ago, but it was only in

Table 11.4
Dosage for calcium-channel blockers.

	Normal daily dose
Dihydropyridines	
Amlodipine	5–10 mg o.d.
Lacidipine	2–6 mg o.d. or b.d.
Nifedipine tablets	10–20 mg b.d. or t.d.s.
Nifedipine LA	30–60 mg o.d.
Verapamil	80–160 mg b.d. or t.d.s.
	Slow release 120–240 mg b.d.
Diltiazem	60–240 mg daily
	Dosage and frequency will depend on formulation

the 1980s that they really came into use as blood pressure-lowering agents. Their exact mode of action in causing peripheral vasodilatation is not understood, but it is likely that by blocking the L-type channels in the cell membrane they cause a reduction in calcium in arteriolar smooth muscle, causing vasodilatation. The CCBs, particularly the dihydropyridines, have also been shown to be natriuretic, and they have a mild 'diuretic' action. Some patients notice nocturia and frequency.

In 1995, several papers were published based on retrospective case control studies that suggested that the use of CCBs was associated with an excess mortality from coronary heart disease, gastrointestinal haemorrhage and a medley of cancers. These findings were not confirmed in several similar studies, and in 1997 the results of the SYST-EUR trial provided reassurance on this point, with no adverse effects on mortality or morbidity from any cause.

There are three major groups of CCBs (Table 11.4):

1. The dihydropyridines, the first of which was nifedipine—there are now a large number of similar drugs.
2. Verapamil, which has a greater negative ionotropic and chronotropic effect on the heart. Although many derivatives of verapamil are being developed, none of them are currently widely used.
3. Diltiazem, which appears to lie between the dihydropyridines and verapamil and has antianginal properties.

Dihydropyridines

These drugs are both peripheral and coronary vasodilators and can be used to treat angina as well as hypertension. However, unlike verapamil, they appear to have no effect on cardiac conduction. The older dihydropyridines are rapidly absorbed, causing a rapid rise in plasma levels that result in the well-known vasodilating side-effects of the dihydropyridines with flushing, headache and dizziness. This was a particular problem with nifedipine capsules, which should no longer be used. These drugs are also short-acting because of fast metabolism in the liver. Large peak/trough variations in the plasma levels cause large variations in blood pressure. Naturally long-acting drugs, such as amlodipine, which have a long half-life, cause fewer vasodilating side-effects because there is a slow rise in plasma levels that reach a steady state after about 7 days of treatment.

The dihydropyridines also cause non-pitting ankle oedema when used in high doses. This is not due to fluid retention as these drugs have diuretic properties. The swelling is due to altered tissue permeability and does not respond to diuretic therapy.

Nifedipine

This was the first dihydropyridine to become available, initially in capsule formulation. The capsule formulation has a rapid onset of action and should no longer be used except in the very rare circumstance of an unconscious patient with hypertensive encephalopathy where intravenous drugs cannot be given. It can cause a very rapid fall in blood pressure, which may be dangerous. Nifedipine tablets are less rapidly absorbed, but are relatively short-acting, so need to be given twice daily. Various attempts have been made to slow down nifedipine absorption, and there are several different slow-release formulations available.

The most effective is the formulation that uses a gastrointestinal transport system (GITS). This gives fairly constant plasma levels over 24 hours, and is therefore the preferable way of giving nifedipine.

Amlodipine

Amlodipine is the only dihydropyridine currently available with a long half-life of at least 36 hours. Steady state plasma levels are reached after about 7–8 days but the drug does not accumulate and there is very little peak/trough change with once-daily dosing. Because of the pharmacokinetics, amlodipine has a slow onset, taking several days to reach full effect. When the drug is stopped, it takes several days for blood pressure to return to pretreatment levels. Amlodipine causes fewer vasodilating effects because of this slow onset, but is as effective as other dihydropyrindines in lowering blood pressure. There is also evidence of a good dose response, so that if 5 mg is not effective the dose can be doubled to 10 mg. However, almost 50% of patients develop ankle oedema on 10 mg daily.

Amlodipine has been called a 'forgiving' drug, as if one single daily dose is omitted blood pressures remain under control. Patients should not be encouraged to miss out their tablets, but amlodipine could be regarded as particularly suitable for non-compliant or 'unreliable' patients.

Other dihydropyridines

There are several other dihydropyridines. Most of them are short-acting and need to be given twice daily. Some are available in slow-release formulations. Felodipine and Lacidipine do appear to be long acting and reasonably free of side-effects.

Indications for dihydropyridines

These drugs are now widely used for the first-line treatment of hypertension. They are particularly effective in older patients, Afro-Caribbeans and patients with severe hypertension. Unlike beta-blockers and diuretics, they have no metabolic effects on cholesterol, potassium or blood sugar. CCBs are widely used in patients with renal failure, where they are effective. They have an additive effect on blood pressure when added to an ACE inhibitor. This is now a very widely used regime in the treatment of more severe hypertension. The dihydropyridines are also effective when used in combination with a beta-blocker, and it has also been reported that beta-blockers reduce the side-effects of nifedipine. Interestingly, when thiazide diuretics are added to a dihydropyridine, there is little further fall in blood pressure, but the metabolic effects of the diuretic persist. Therefore, in patients treated with dihydropyridines alone, there is no point in adding a diuretic.

Side-effects

There are two well recognised side-effects of dihydropyridines (Table 11.5). The first is headache, flushing and dizziness, mainly due to a rapid rise in the plasma levels with short-acting agents. These effects can be minimised by using amlodipine or a slow-release formulation of a short-acting drug. The second side-effect of dihydropyridines that occurs is a shift of sodium and water into the legs owing to a change in capillary haemodynamics. This may cause ankle oedema, particularly in those who have a tendency to develop swollen ankles. With the initiation of therapy, there may often be transient oedema, or discomfort in the legs, though this improves after a few days.

Table 11.5

Side-effects of dihydropyridines and verapamil.

Facial flushing
Headaches
Ankle oedema
Nocturia
Constipation
Gum hyperplasia

However, if the oedema persists, a reduction in dose should be tried. If this does not help then it is better to switch to a different form of therapy. An important but under-reported side-effect of the dihydropyridines is nocturia, particularly in middle-aged men. Gum hyperplasia is not uncommon with all the CCBs, and particularly with nifedipine and amlodipine.

Verapamil

Verapamil was originally introduced in the late 1960s as a beta-blocker and was used intravenously as an antiarrhythmic agent. Subsequently, it became clear that it was a calcium antagonist and an effective blood pressure-lowering drug. However, there were concerns when patients who were receiving a beta-blocker were given intravenous verapamil, as it precipitated sinus arrest in some patients. In view of this, it is best not to use oral verapamil with a beta-blocker.

Like many of the other CCBs, verapamil is rapidly metabolised and in conventional formulation needs to be given twice or three times daily. Many slow-release preparations have been developed that vary from country to country, particularly as verapamil is now off patent.

Side-effects

The major side-effect of verapamil is constipation. This occurs particularly when higher doses are used. It can be largely overcome by patients consuming a high-fibre diet. In some patients the constipation may be so severe that verapamil has to be stopped. Verapamil should not be used in combination with a beta-blocker unless there is some very good reason to do so. However, it is additive to an ACE inhibitor, and even the addition of a diuretic may have some extra effect on blood pressure. Verapamil has been shown to be as effective as beta-blockers in secondary prevention following a myocardial infarction.

Diltiazem

This is an effective blood pressure-lowering drug that can also be used for angina pectoris. It has less negative inotropic effects than verapamil, but slightly more than the dihydropyridines. Like nifedipine it is rapidly metabolised and, in conventional formulation, needs to be given twice or three times a day. A variety of slow-release forms of diltiazem have become available.

Side-effects

Diltiazem causes fewer vasodilating symptoms and probably slightly less oedema than the dihydropyridines and less constipation than verapamil. As with the other CCBs, the side-effects of diltiazem are dose-related.

Indications for diltiazem

Diltiazem is widely used in some countries as first-line therapy for hypertension. It is additive to ACE inhibitors. In view of its slightly negative ionotropic and chronotropic effect, there was some concern about its use in combination with beta-blockers. The addition of a diuretic to diltiazem may have a slightly greater blood pressure-lowering effect than adding a diuretic to the dihydropyridines.

Table 11.6
Dosage for ACE inhibitors.

	Normal daily dose
Captopril	12.5–50 mg b.d. or t.d.s.
Enalapril	2.5–20 mg o.d. or b.d.
Fosinopril	10–20 g o.d. or b.d.
Lisinopril	2.5–20 mg o.d. or b.d.
Perindopril	2–4 mg o.d. or b.d.
Quinapril	5–20 mg o.d. or b.d.
Ramipril	1.25–5 mg o.d. or b.d.
Trandolapril	1–2 mg o.d. or b.d.

ACE INHIBITORS

These drugs were specifically designed to block the enzyme that is responsible for converting the inactive peptide angiotensin I to the active and powerful vasoconstrictor angiotensin II. The first inhibitor was found in snake venom and, from this, an injectable peptide was developed. Subsequently, compounds that could be taken orally were synthesised. Captopril was the first of this new class of compounds. Since then a large number of other ACE inhibitors have been developed (Table 11.6). In general, this class of drugs is remarkably well tolerated.

There are no major differences between the ACE inhibitors apart from two factors. Some ACE inhibitors are taken as 'prodrugs', which are metabolised to the active compound in the liver. Enalapril and perindopril are 'prodrugs' and, in theory at least, they may be less effective in patients with hepatic impairment. They may, however, be less prone to cause first-dose hypotension. The other important difference is in the pharmacokinetics. Some ACE inhibitors, particularly captopril, are rapidly metabolised and are short-acting.

Mode of action

It is now realised that the renin–angiotensin system is important in the control of blood pressure. Circulating angiotensin II has multiple actions with direct vasoconstriction of arterioles, sodium and water retention both directly and through aldosterone, as well as stimulation of the sympathetic nervous system. Unsurprisingly, therefore, when the formation of angiotensin II is blocked by an ACE inhibitor, blood pressure falls. There is controversy about the importance of local non-circulating renin–angiotensin systems. It is clear, however, that when angiotensin II is generated in the tissues, the renin that is available is derived from the kidney. ACE inhibitors may also prevent the breakdown of bradykinin, a potential vasodilator. However, it remains unclear how important this effect is, and the role of bradykinin has been exaggerated. Perhaps more importantly, the ACE inhibitors, through angiotensin II, may influence prostaglandin metabolism and this may contribute to the reduction in blood pressure.

Side-effects (Table 11.7)

The commonest side-effect of ACE inhibitors is an irritating dry cough, which may occur in up to 15% of patients. It may be particularly bad at night. There is no evidence that any one ACE inhibitor causes less cough than another. There are some suggestions that it is more common in middle-aged females, non-smokers and possibly in Chinese people. The mechanism of the cough is unknown. In some cases, a reduction in dose or a switch to another ACE inhibitor can be tried. Usually this has little effect and the drug has to be stopped. Many patients may not associate the cough with the treatment, so it is important to question them and their partners. Cough is a very common symptom and ACE inhibitors should not unnecessarily be withdrawn unless there clearly is an association. The cough may take up to 6 weeks to abate after discontinuation. If in doubt, the ACE inhibitor can always be restarted to see if the cough recurs.

Occasionally, ACE inhibitors cause recurrent or acute angioedema with swelling of the lips, tongue, face and upper respiratory tract. Laryngeal oedema can lead to respiratory obstruction and death. This side-effect occurs in one in 4000 patients, but is commoner in patients of African origin.

ACE inhibitors can occasionally cause a deterioration in renal function. This is likely to occur in patients with renal artery stenosis, particularly if there is narrowing of both arteries or narrowing of the artery supplying a single functioning kidney. ACE inhibitors should not be used in these patients unless there are exceptional circumstances. Renal artery stenosis is more common than previously thought, and occurs in many older patients who are cigarette smokers, particularly if they already have peripheral vascular or coronary artery disease. In such

Table 11.7
Side-effects of ACE inhibitors.

Dry irritating cough
Deterioration of renal function in renal artery stenosis
Angioedema
Hypotension if prior volume depletion

patients, if an ACE inhibitor is being given then renal function must be checked before and 1 or 2 weeks after starting therapy. If there is a deterioration in renal function this strongly suggests that the patients have renal artery stenosis. Care should also be taken in patients who already have renal impairment or who are volume-depleted, particularly after large doses of diuretics.

ACE inhibitors, particularly captopril, may occasionally cause a skin rash, which is characteristically morbilliform. More rarely, captopril may cause a loss of taste. However, with the lower doses of ACE inhibitors that are now used, these effects are extremely rare.

Because of the reduction of circulating angiotensin and aldosterone levels, ACE inhibitors tend to cause a small rise in plasma potassium concentration. This may be marginally beneficial if these drugs are being given in combination with a diuretic. In patients with renal impairment, dangerous hyperkalaemia may be encountered, particularly if potassium-sparing diuretics are also being used.

The major advantage of the ACE inhibitors over other classes of antihypertensive drugs is their relative lack of side-effects. Many patients feel entirely normal, and do not complain of the subtle and insidious side-effects seen with the beta-blockers.

Additional effects of ACE inhibitors

There is now good evidence that ACE inhibitors have beneficial effects in patients with both diabetic and non-diabetic nephropathy. This is related to their vasodilating effects on the post-glomerular efferent arterioles, reducing intraglomerular pressure. Renal failure may be delayed and, occasionally, renal function may be improved.

The ACE inhibitors have also been shown to be superior to other drugs at reducing left ventricular hypertrophy (LVH) in severely hypertensive patients. This effect appears to be independent of the blood pressure-lowering properties. Furthermore, ACE inhibitors have been shown to prolong life in patients with heart failure or left ventricular systolic dysfunction following a heart attack. More recently, evidence has emerged that ACE inhibitors may delay the progression of diabetic retinopathy.

The blood pressure-lowering effect of the ACE inhibitors largely depends on the plasma levels of angiotensin II and renin, which in turn depends on salt intake. The effectiveness of these drugs is markedly increased if patients restrict their salt intake. Similarly, diuretics are additive to ACE inhibitors and low doses of diuretics are very effective. All CCBs are additive to ACE inhibitors. However, the additional effect of beta-blockers with ACE inhibitors is small, and this combination is not recommended.

Differences between ACE inhibitors

Captopril, the first ACE inhibitor, is rapidly absorbed and has a short duration of action. This may be useful for test dosing whilst initiating ACE inhibitor therapy, especially in patients with heart failure. However, in the routine treatment of hypertension, captopril needs to be given at least twice daily and more frequently in some patients. The other ACE inhibitors are longer acting and claims have been made that they can be given once daily, although in our experience this is not always so. When given once daily, there may be large peak/trough effects with the ACE inhibitors. Blood pressure should be checked before patients take the next dose to make sure it remains controlled throughout 24 hours. In many patients it may be better to give a lower dose of the longer-acting drugs twice daily rather than a high dose once daily. Most ACE inhibitors are excreted by the kidney and, depending on the exact mode of excretion and whether some of the metabolites are active, they may accumulate in patients with renal impairment. Claims have been made that those drugs that are excreted mainly by the liver may be safer in these patients.

Enalapril is the most widely used ACE inhibitor. It is a prodrug that is converted in the liver to its active form enalaprilat. It is longer acting than captopril so can be given in some patients once daily. Lisinopril, a lysine analogue of enalapril, is directly absorbed and acts directly. It is excreted by the kidney and thus may accumulate in renal disease. It appears to be slightly longer acting than enalapril. Trandolopril and perindopril are also relatively long-acting.

ANGIOTENSIN-RECEPTOR ANTAGONISTS (THE SARTANS)

Recently introduced, this is a new class of drug that specifically blocks the receptors for angiotensin II (Table 11.8). This represents a new way of blocking the renin–angiotensin system and has already

Table 11.8

Dosage of angiotensin-receptor antagonists.

	Normal daily dose
Losartan	50–100 mg o.d.
Valsartan	80–160 mg o.d.
Irbesartan	150–300 mg o.d.
Telmisartan*	20–160 mg o.d.
Eprosartan*	600–800 mg o.d.
Candesartan	8–16 mg o.d.

*The final dosage of these drugs when launched will be within this range.

been proven to be effective in the treatment of high blood pressure, as well as heart failure. The major advantage of this new class of compounds is that they appear to be free, so far, of major side-effects.

Angiotensin II exerts its effect on tissues through specific receptors. The first compounds to be developed in the mid-1970s were peptide antagonists, which were used to investigate the possibility of blocking the renin system in this way. They had to be given intravenously and had the disadvantage of some agonist activity because they tended to stimulate the angiotensin II receptors when circulating levels of angiotensin II were low.

Over the last decade, potent, orally absorbed non-peptide drugs that are more powerful inhibitors of the angiotensin II receptors have been developed. With these receptor antagonists, it has become clear that there are at least two classes of angiotensin II receptors. The AT1 receptor appears to be responsible for nearly all the physiological actions of angiotensin II. The role of the AT2 receptors remains ill-defined, although one possible function is that they may inhibit cell growth in some tissues.

There are now at least six different angiotensin-receptor antagonists on the market, or about to be launched. They are all specific AT1-receptor antagonists and do not block the AT2 receptors. The first 'sartan' to be developed, losartan, and subsequently a large series of compounds, are all extremely effective in blocking the AT1 receptors for angiotensin II.

Losartan

Losartan is a relatively weak angiotensin II-receptor antagonist, but it is converted into a long-acting and active metabolite that specifically blocks the AT1 receptors. This metabolite is responsible for the long duration of action. A large number of clinical studies have now shown that losartan given 50 or 100 mg once daily, is as effective as other antihypertensive drugs, including enalapril, the dihydropyridines and the beta-blockers. Losartan, like all the drugs that block the renin–angiotensin system, is particularly effective if patients have already reduced their salt intake, and has an additive effect with diuretics and calcium antagonists. Losartan, like all the sartans, is remarkably well-tolerated and in studies so far has no more side-effects than placebo. Importantly, in a carefully controlled double-blind study, in patients who had previously developed a cough with lisinopril and were re-challenged, losartan did not cause a cough. This has also been found with all other angiotensin II-receptor antagonists. These trials, therefore, demonstrate that none of the angiotensin II-receptor antagonists are associated with cough, unlike the ACE inhibitors, and there are also, so far, no reports of angioedema.

An important study in mild heart failure in the elderly compared losartan 50 mg daily, against captopril 50 mg three times daily (the 'ELITE' study). This showed that losartan was as good as captopril in the control of heart failure, and there was a significant trend for a greater reduction in all-cause mortality with losartan, in particular with a reduction in sudden death. Further, larger studies are ongoing to see if there are other advantages with the angiotensin II-receptor antagonists over ACE inhibitors in both heart failure and renal disease.

The newer sartans

Several other angiotensin II-receptor antagonists are now on the market or about to be launched. These include valsartan, candesartan, irbesartan, telmisartan and eprosartan. All have been shown to be as effective as other antihypertensive drugs, and some have been shown to be additive to salt restriction, diuretics and calcium antagonists.

Studies with valsartan and candesartan in comparison with losartan have claimed that they may be more effective, though whether this is due to a longer length of action, differences in dosing schedule, or a real increase in effectiveness is not clear. All these angiotensin II-receptor antagonists have been shown to be remarkably free of side-effects. Candesartan has been shown in a well-controlled study in resistant hypertension to be effective on its own and, in particular, to be effective at controlling blood pressure in combination with the dihydropyridine, amlodipine, and a thiazide diuretic.

As with the ACE inhibitors, the angiotensin II-receptor antagonists should be used with caution in patients with renal artery stenosis. They may cause a deterioration in renal function in these patients, although this may be less likely with the sartans than with ACE inhibitors. All angiotensin II-receptor antagonists, through inhibition of the negative feedback of angiotensin II on the juxtaglomerular apparatus, cause an increase in renin release and a rise in circulating levels of angiotensin II. Initially, there was concern that this would cause excessive stimulation of the AT2 receptors which were not blocked by the angiotensin receptor antagonist. Recent work has suggested that these receptors may be important in promoting cell growth and that the increased levels of angiotensin II may inhibit cell growth, which in certain circumstances could be seen as an advantage. As yet, the relevance of these findings to man are not clear. Importantly, although there is no current evidence of adverse effects through not inhibiting the AT2 receptors.

Because of their effectiveness in lowering blood pressure and their lack of side-effects coupled with the findings in the 'ELITE' study of equivalence or a slight advantage over captopril in heart failure, the angiotensin II-receptor antagonists are becoming one of the major new classes of drugs for the treatment of hypertension. Outcome studies are ongoing and, given their advantages over ACE inhibitors in not causing angioedema, cough or any other side-effect, angiotensin II receptor antagonists are likely to be widely used in the treatment of high blood pressure in the future.

ALPHA₁-RECEPTOR ANTAGONISTS

This class of drug was not initially popular because of the complexity of dosage regimes and the high frequency of side-effects. However, recently, two longer acting

Table 11.9
Dosage for alpha-adrenoceptor blockers and combined alpha and beta-receptor antagonists.

	Normal daily dose
Alpha-blockers	
Doxazosin	1–16 mg o.d.
Prazosin	0.5–5 mg t.d.s.
Terazosin	1–20 mg o.d.
Alpha- and beta-receptor antagonists	
Labetalol	100–400 mg b.d.

alpha-blockers have been developed, doxazosin and terazosin, which are fairly well tolerated. This has led to renewed interest in the alpha-blockers (Table 11.9).

Phenoxybenzamine and phentolamine

Phenoxybenzamine is only used in patients with phaeochromocytoma, where it is effective. The starting dose is 10 mg twice daily, but much larger doses are needed until blood pressure is controlled. Once phenoxybenzamine is introduced, a beta-blocker can be added to control the heart rate if this is increased. Phenoxybenzamine invariably causes some postural hypotension and problems with ejaculation.

Phentolamine is a very short-acting alpha-blocker available only by intravenous injection. It can be used in hypertensive crises in patients with phaeochromocytoma, rebound hypertension following clonidine withdrawal or reactions to the monoamine-oxidase inhibitors.

Prazosin

This is a short-acting alpha-blocker, which has to be taken three times daily. Patients occasionally develop 'first-dose hypotension', so it is usually recommended that the first dose of 1 mg should be taken at night in bed. We are of the opinion that this drug should no longer be used.

Doxazosin and terazosin

These are both longer acting alpha-blockers, which can be given once daily. They appear to have fewer side-effects than the short-acting alpha-blockers, such as prazosin, and are effective in lowering blood pressure. In view of the fact that they do cause slight falls in cholesterol, claims have been made that they may have advantages in the long-term treatment of hypertension, but these have yet to be clearly demonstrated. They are claimed to be additive to diuretics, beta-blockers, calcium antagonists and ACE inhibitors. When combined with other drugs they can cause postural drops in blood pressure; this should be borne in mind and standing blood pressures should be measured. First dose hypotension does occur with doxazocin.

Alpha-blockers affect the alpha receptors at the bladder neck. In men this can lead to some relief from the symptoms of benign prostate hypertrophy and also some improvement in sexual function. In women, however, alpha-blockers can cause or aggravate stress incontinence.

Other alpha-blockers

Indoramine has been marketed both for the treatment of hypertension as well as the relief of prostatic symptoms. We do not recommend it for hypertension. Alfuzosin and tamsulosin are also alpha-blockers used exclusively for prostatism. Both can cause 'first-dose' effects not unlike prazocin and should be used with caution in hypertensive patients.

COMBINED ALPHA- AND BETA-RECEPTOR ANTAGONISTS

Alpha-blockers and beta-blockers have been used together to treat hypertension. Only one drug combines both alpha and beta blockade.

Labetalol

Labetalol is both a beta-blocker and a weak alpha-blocker when taken orally. However, when given intravenously, it has much greater alpha-blocking properties. Intravenous labetalol is sometimes used in hypertensive emergencies. When given orally, its long-term effect on blood pressure is similar to that of beta-blockers, except when very high doses are given, when the alpha-blocking property is then apparent, particularly in causing postural hypotension. Labetalol also appears to have more side-effects than many beta-blockers, particularly causing itchiness of the scalp. Several studies have been done on hypertension in pregnancy, and it has been shown to be useful in this situation. It is no longer widely used otherwise.

CENTRAL ALPHA$_2$-RECEPTOR AGONISTS

The central alpha-receptor agonists were first introduced in the 1960s, and became, in many countries, the most commonly used antihypertensive drugs after the diuretics. This class of drugs includes methyldopa and clonidine. Exactly how methyldopa works is not clear. It was originally thought that it inhibited the enzyme converting dopa to dopamine. However, more recent research has shown that both methyldopa and clonidine lower blood pressure by central alpha$_2$ receptor stimulation. Whilst they are effective in lowering blood pressure, and are additive to many of the other antihypertensive regimes, their side-effects, in comparison with the more modern drugs, are such that most physicians no longer use them.

Methyldopa

Methyldopa is an effective antihypertensive drug but has a large number of side-effects. Nearly all patients notice they feel sleepy, particularly during the first few weeks, and many feel debilitated or depressed. This may become apparent when patients stop long-term methyldopa and frequently report that they feel much better. It can cause depression, and it may also cause impotence or failure of ejaculation. Several drug reactions can occur with methyldopa. These include liver dysfunction, a positive direct Coomb's test and, more rarely, haemolytic anaemia and drug fever. Many patients who started on methyldopa in the 1960s and 1970s have learned to live with their side-effects. Our view is that all patients receiving methyldopa should be offered a trial of alternative therapy, even though they may not have realised how their life was being impaired.

The only indication for methyldopa is in pregnancy-related hypertension, where it appears to be safe. There are no reports of postnatal depression related to methyldopa therapy, but this possibility must be born in mind.

Clonidine

This is very similar to methyldopa. It is an effective antihypertensive drug but causes many of the same side-effects such as sedation and nasal stuffiness. However, unlike methyldopa, it does not cause hepatic or haematological problems. More worrying is the rebound hypertension that occurs when clonidine is withdrawn. This is particularly dangerous if patients are also receiving a beta-blocker, when the omission of even one dose of clonidine may result in a hypertensive crisis. Because of this, and its side-effect profile, clonidine should no longer be used. Where patients are stopping clonidine, it is important to withdraw the beta-blocker first and to substitute a calcium antagonist. The dose of clonidine should gradually be reduced and blood pressure should be closely monitored.

IMIDAZOLINE-RECEPTOR AGONISTS

This is a new class of antihypertensive drugs that shares some of the actions of clonidine on the newly described central imidazoline receptors. This means there should be fewer central nervous system side-effects like sedation and depression. Rilmenidine is now available in some countries and moxonidine has been launched in the UK.

Moxonidine

Clinical trial evidence suggests this is a safe and effective antihypertensive drug with few side-effects, although there are early reports of disturbance of liver enzymes. It should prove additive to all the other drug classes, and its use so far has largely been confined to severe resistant hypertension. The dose is 200–400 µg once daily.

DIRECT-ACTING VASODILATORS

The direct arteriolar vasodilators (Table 11.10), such as hydralazine, cause a decrease in peripheral vascular tone but have the disadvantage of causing a reflex activation of the sympathetic nervous system and an increase in heart rate. This increase in sympathetic activity and the resultant rise in angiotensin II levels also account for the retention of sodium and water that occurs. However, when given in combination with a beta-blocker and diuretic, side-effects are minimised, and this was a widely used combination in the 1970s. Worldwide, hydralazine is still frequently used, usually in combination with reserpine and a thiazide, but it is now hardly ever used in the UK.

Hydralazine

Hydralazine has a direct effect on smooth muscle cells in the peripheral arterioles and only a small effect on veins. It is largely metabolised by the liver. On its own, it is not very effective at lowering blood pressure because of reflex sympathetic stimulation.

Table 11.10
Dosage for peripheral vasodilators.

	Normal daily dose
Hydralazine	25–50 mg b.d.
Minoxidil	2.5–20 mg b.d.

Many patients develop symptoms of peripheral vasodilatation, including headaches, flushing and palpitations. This is alleviated to some extent by adding a beta-blocker. Some patients develop a lupus-like syndrome with arthritis, pyrexia and general malaise. This usually occurs at higher doses or in patients who metabolise the drug slowly (slow acetylators). It is likely that this syndrome is more common than has been recognised previously because the symptoms may be mild.

Minoxidil and diazoxide

Minoxidil is the most potent vasodilator known. It is thought to act in a similar way to hydralazine, and again causes reflex sympathetic stimulation, leading to tachycardia and sodium and water retention. It also causes hirsuites and, in view of this side-effect, it was largely reserved for men with very severe, uncontrolled hypertension. With the advent of the calcium antagonists and ACE inhibitors the need for minoxidil has diminished. Nevertheless, in patients who are resistant to all other therapy, it still has a role. The major problem with the drug is oedema, which is prevented by the use of frusemide, often in large doses. Like hydralazine, it is best used in combination with a beta-blocker.

Diazoxide, like minoxidil, is a powerful direct-acting vasodilator. It is no longer used because it may cause glucose intolerance or even frank diabetes. This side-effect is due to the fact that it is chemically related to the thiazide diuretics. However, unlike the thiazides, it causes fluid retention. The only role for diazoxide is in the management of hypertensive emergencies where intravenous therapy is considered necessary. However, if large doses are given rapidly there may be a precipitate and dangerous fall in blood pressure leading to cerebral or myocardial infarction. Diazoxide can be given by infusion or by mini-bolus injections starting at an initial dose of 50 mg (see Chapter 12).

OTHER ANTIHYPERTENSIVE DRUGS

Rauwolfia alkaloids

These drugs were widely used in the 1950s and 1960s and have both central and peripheral effects on noradrenaline release. Reserpine was the most widely used drug. However, it was found to cause sedation, depression and even suicide. Nevertheless, at low doses, 0.1–0.2 mg, given at night and combined with a diuretic, it is effective. Because it is very cheap this remains a widely used combination in many developing countries.

Post-adrenergic blockers (guanethidine, bethanidine and debrisoquine)

All these drugs have serious side-effects, including postural hypotension, exercise-induced hypotension, failure of ejaculation, impotence and, rarely, severe diarrhoea. These drugs should therefore no longer be used and patients already on them should be changed to more modern treatment.

FURTHER READING

Beevers DG, Sleight P. Short acting dihydropyridine (vasodilating) calcium channel blockers for hypertension: is there a risk? *Br Med J* 1996; **312**: 1183–5.

Lyons D, Petrie JC, Reid JL. Drug treatment: present and future. *Br Med Bull* 1994; **50**: 472–93.

Materson BJ, Reda DJ, Cushman WC, *et al.* Single-drug therapy for hypertension in men: a comparison of six antihypertensive agents with placebo. *N Engl J Med* 1993; **328**: 914–21.

Messerli FH, Weber MA, Brunner HR. Angiotensin II receptor inhibition. A new therapeutic principle. *Arch Intern Med* 1996; **156**: 1957–65

Morris STW, Reid JL. Moxonidine: a review. *J Hum Hypertens* 1997; **11**: 629–35

Neaton JD, Grimm RH, Prineas RJ, *et al.* Treatment of mild hypertension study (TOMHS): final results. *JAMA* 1993; **270**: 713–24.

12 SCHEMES FOR REDUCING BLOOD PRESSURE

BACKGROUND

There is a large variety of drugs that lower blood pressure with different mechanisms of action. New types of drugs and/or new formulations or combinations of existing agents are continuously being developed. Often, by the time definitive evidence of the usefulness of a group of drugs in preventing the complications of hypertension has become available, new products have been developed that may have advantages and fewer side-effects. It is not surprising, therefore, that there is disagreement between experts on which drugs or combinations of drugs are best for individual patients.

Up to recently, the treatment of most forms of high blood pressure was relatively simple. Patients were started on either a beta-blocker or a thiazide diuretic and if one drug was insufficient, the two were used in combination and then further drugs were added in sequentially. This so-called 'step-care' approach has now been abandoned, as it is clear that individual patients respond to different drugs in different ways, and many patients develop side-effects, particularly from the beta-blockers, which are rapidly declining in popularity.

In our view, all the available antihypertensive drugs can be regarded as candidates for first-line therapy, with the choice based on the patient's characteristics. This is sometimes described as the 'tailored-care' approach to antihypertensive treatment.

WHAT IS THE LEVEL OF BLOOD PRESSURE TO AIM FOR?

The objective of antihypertensive therapy is to reduce the diastolic blood pressure to below 90 mmHg and the systolic pressure at least to below 160 mmHg. Epidemiological evidence would suggest that blood pressure should be reduced even further and in the USA, treatment guidelines now state that the systolic pressure should be reduced to below 140 mmHg. The Hypertension Optimal Treatment (HOT) trial (see Chapter 9), published in 1998, strongly suggests that this is correct as in the 18790 treated hypertensives in the study, the 'optimum' blood pressure at follow-up was 139/83 mmHg.

There is reliable evidence that the outlook for a hypertensive patient is more closely related to the quality of blood pressure control than to the height of the blood pressure in the first place. Mild hypertensive patients with poor control have a worse prognosis than severe hypertensives with good blood pressure control (Fig 9.8).

The more severe the hypertension before treatment, the greater the risk of death, but greater too are the benefits of treatment. In general, the same drugs are used whatever the level of blood pressure, but in patients with severe hypertension there is a greater urgency to reduce blood pressure and less time to establish the best approach for the individual patient. However, the urgency of treatment is commonly overstressed and, apart from cases with hypertensive encephalopathy, gross hypertensive left ventricular failure or hypertension associated with aortic dissection, there is rarely a need to reduce blood pressure over minutes or even hours. Even in patients with accelerated hypertension, blood pressure should be lowered only over 24–48 hours and, during that period, it should not be reduced to normal levels. Over-rapid blood pressure reduction in patients with severe hypertension can cause both strokes and heart attacks.

BLOOD PRESSURE-LOWERING REGIMES

Non-pharmacological blood pressure reduction

All patients should be instructed on non-pharmacological ways in which blood pressure may be lowered (see Chapter 10). Non-pharmacological treatment is most often stressed only to patients with mild hypertension, but it is also effective in combination with drug treatment in more severe cases. All patients with hypertension should be instructed on salt restriction and, where relevant, weight loss and moderation of alcohol intake.

First-line antihypertensive drug therapy

There are now six classes of first-line antihypertensive drugs. These are:

(i)   thiazide diuretics
(ii)   beta-blockers
(iii)   calcium-channel blockers (CCBs)
(iv)   ACE inhibitors
(v)   angiotensin-receptor antagonists
(vi)   alpha-blockers.

It is our view that any of these drugs can be used as first-line therapy. However, some physicians adopt a more conservative approach on the grounds that long-term outcome trials have only been conducted so far with diuretics and beta-blockers, so these drugs should be used first. Only when they fail, or cause side-effects, should the other classes of compounds be used. We feel, particularly in the light of the results of the SYST-EUR trial where calcium-channel blockers with or without ACE inhibitors were effective in preventing heart attacks and strokes, that this approach is now obsolete. The guiding principal is to control blood pressure and minimise side-effects using the most appropriate drugs for individual patients.

GUIDELINES

Several organisations, including the British Hypertension Society (BHS), published

Table 12.1
A guide to blood pressure treatment.

(a) Non-pharmacological

All patients   (i)   Salt restriction
                        (ii)   Weight control
                        (iii)   Alcohol moderation

(b) First-line drugs

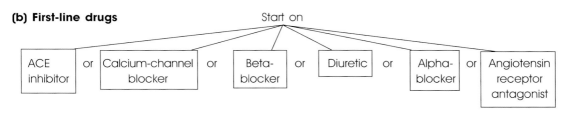

guidelines for the treatment of hypertension in 1993. In general they tended to be somewhat conservative and were controversial at the time. The publication in 1997 of the SYST-EUR trial and the success of the angiotensin-receptor antagonists means that some of these guidelines are now seriously out of date. Similarly, the resuts of the HOT trial must influence guidelines committees in their deliberations on future guidelines.

Of all the guidelines, probably those from New Zealand are the most sensible as they do draw attention to the concept of absolute risk. The clinician should consider what are the chances that a patient will sustain a heart attack or stroke and by what amount can this be reduced. The first part of the question depends on the patient's age, smoking status, serum cholesterol levels, as well as the height of the blood pressure. The answer to the second question is easier; antihypertensive treatment reduces stroke by 40% and heart attack by 20%.

Perhaps the final question the clinician should ask himself is what drug would he choose to take if he himself was the patient.

We suspect that beta-blockers and thiazide diuretics would not figure so prominently if this approach were to be more frequently applied.

THE FIRST STEP

In this section we outline the six classes of compounds and the various indications and contraindications for them as first-line therapy, as well as our preferred choices of treatment in each class (Table 12.1).

Diuretics

There are no basic differences between the many thiazide diuretics. If this group of drugs is used then the best option is to prescribe the cheapest, at a low dose. The thiazides have a flat dose response on blood pressure so little is achieved by using bigger doses in terms of blood pressure reduction. However, metabolic side-effects are greater with higher doses. It is our practice to use either bendrofluazide in a single daily dose of 1.25 or 2.5 mg or hydrochlorothiazide 12.5–25 mg daily as this minimises the clinical and metabolic side-effects. Studies in elderly patients have clearly demonstrated that the thiazides reduce not only strokes, but also coronary heart disease.

Thiazide diuretics are most useful in:

- black patients
- elderly patients
- patients with mild or incipient heart failure.

In general, they are best avoided in:

- patients with NIDDM
- patients with hyperlipidaemia
- pregnancy
- patients with gout
- sexually active males.

One of the major side-effects of thiazide diuretics is male impotence, and they should be discontinued in men complaining of this, as well as in patients who develop hyperglycaemia or hyperlipidaemia.

Patients receiving diuretics of any type should have their serum electrolytes checked after about 2 months, and annually thereafter. It is not our practice to prescribe potassium supplements, but an increase in dietary potassium is advised. Combined diuretic and potassium tablets should not be used as they only contain small amounts of potassium.

If the serum potassium falls then the potassium-sparing diuretics (amiloride or triamterene) may be added. The addition of a beta-blocker or an ACE inhibitor to a low dose of a thiazide diuretic also blunts the fall in serum potassium. Patients on long-term thiazide therapy should have occasional checks of their urine or blood for

glucose, and their serum lipid levels should also be checked. If marked hypokalaemia develops with the use of thiazide diuretics in suitably low dosage, a diagnosis of underlying primary hyperaldosteronism should be considered.

Beta-blockers

The differences between the many beta-blockers are not great. Nearly all of them can be given in once-daily dosage regimes, and the contraindications are well recognised. As with the thiazide diuretics, it is generally advisable to use the lowest dose, although this may have to be given twice daily.

Beta-blockers are most useful in:

- younger patients
- anxious patients
- angina pectoris
- patients who have had a myocardial infarction.

Beta-blockers should be avoided in:

- patients with asthma or a history of asthma
- 'brittle' insulin-requiring diabetics
- any patients with peripheral vascular disease
- Raynaud's syndrome
- second and third degree heart block
- patients with heart failure
- energetic patients.

While the beta-blockers are effective drugs, they cause a reduction in exercise tolerance with a feeling of heaviness in the legs on climbing stairs or running. The other major side-effect is a subtle change in mentation, with a lack of drive and vigour, often noticed by the spouse or work colleagues but only apparent to the patient when the beta-blocker is stopped.

In the outcome trials, the beta-blockers were less effective compared with the thiazides at preventing strokes and had little or no effect on coronary heart disease. In addition they are not particularly effective in older patients at lowering blood pressure. For this reason their use is declining and we do not recommend them for routine first-line therapy.

Calcium-channel blockers

There are some differences between the CCBs. The dihydropyridines, such as amlodipine and nifedipine, do not slow the heart, whilst verapamil and diltiazem not only cause vasodilation, but also slow the heart rate.

CCBs are most useful in:

- older patients
- black patients
- patients with peripheral vascular disease
- patients with cerebrovascular disease
- patients with angina pectoris.

Verapamil should be avoided in:

- patients with cardiac failure
- patients with heart block
- patients receiving a beta-blocker.

Short-acting dihydropyridines (e.g. nifedipine) should be avoided in:

- unstable angina
- recent myocardial infarction.

One major disadvantage in the past was that the CCBs had a short half-life and this necessitated twice or, in many, three-times-daily therapy. Amlodipine is the only truly long-acting CCB, but the others are available in slow-release formulations, which means they do not have to be given so often. Care, however, needs to be taken with each of these formulations as not all of them are as effective as their manufacturers may claim. The CCBs have the advantage of not causing subtle side-effects, particularly on mentation. However, the short-acting dihydropyridines cause flushing and headaches and the long-acting ones cause gravity-dependent but diuretic-resistant oedema. Verapamil in particular, but also all CCBs, may cause constipation. All these side-effects are dose-related. All CCBs, and particularly nifedipine and amlodipine, cause gum hypertrophy.

ACE inhibitors

This group of drugs has few serious side effects. However, they can cause cough in up to 15% of patients. Acute angioedema, which may be life-threatening with laryngeal oedema, occurs in 1 patient in 4000, and is four times commoner in patients of African origin.

Apart from their length of action and frequency of dosage, it is doubtful whether there are any major differences between the ACE inhibitors when used in the correct dosage. ACE inhibitors are particularly useful in:

- younger patients
- patients with all grades of heart failure
- patients who develop side-effects with other drugs
- diabetic hypertensive patients.
- hypertension with non-diabetic nephropathy.

ACE inhibitors should be used with great care in:

- renal artery stenosis

- patients with extensive atheromatous disease
- fluid-depleted patients, especially those receiving a loop diuretic such as frusemide.

ACE inhibitors should be avoided in:

- pregnancy
- premenopausal women who may become pregnant.

Captopril, the first ACE inhibitor, was short acting, needing a three-times-daily dosage regime to avoid large peak/trough differences. It is better, therefore, to use a longer-acting ACE inhibitor such as enalapril or lisinopril. However, in some patients it may be better to give a low dose twice daily rather than a higher dose once a day, as some ACE inhibitors currently available wear off within 24 hours after the last dose.

Trandolopril and perindopril do appear to be genuinely long acting and can be given once daily.

Alpha₁–blockers

The first alpha-blockers had severe side-effects, particularly causing postural hypotension. However, the long-acting selective alpha₁-blockers, doxazosin and terazosin are effective in lowering blood pressure and lack the side-effects of their predecessors. They also have the advantage of causing a small reduction in serum cholesterol levels and may improve sexual function.

Angiotensin-receptor antagonists

This group of drugs has only been available since 1995, but they have proved safe and effective. They have been used in more than 2 000 000 patients worldwide. They can, therefore, be considered to be suitable for first-line therapy, or as alternative first-line drugs in patients who cannot tolerate the ACE inhibitors.

Other antihypertensive drugs

The centrally acting antihypertensive drugs such as clonidine, methyldopa and reserpine should not be used as first-line therapy in any patient. Their major side-effects of sedation and depression mean that they should no longer be used except in pregnancy (see Chapter 16). The adrenergic blockers, guanethidine, bethanidine and debrisoquine, should no longer be used, and the directly acting vasodilators such as hydralazine, minoxidil and diazoxide should not be used as first-line therapy. It is our view that when patients are encountered taking such drugs, even if blood pressure is well controlled, it may be well worth switching them to more modern drugs as they may feel considerably better.

Moxonidine, the new centrally acting agent, may occasionally be used as a first-line drug if all the others have caused problems.

FAILURE OF FIRST-LINE THERAPY

If the first drug does not lower blood pressure sufficiently, there are three options. One is to change to another first-line drug, another is to add in a second drug and the third is to escalate the dose. The last option is the least desirable as it frequently leads to drug-related side-effects. If side-effects do occur then a second drug should be tried. Some clinicians suggest that all the drugs should be tried as initial therapy before adding in a second drug.

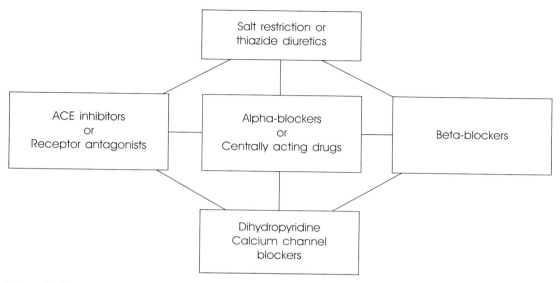

Figure 12.1

A system for the choice of add-on therapies in hypertension.

Clearly, a balance has to be struck between what is practical for the doctor and patient, and what results in the best control of the blood pressure with the patient remaining completely well.

Another suggestion, which has not received enough attention, is that when two additive drugs are combined, lower doses can be used, which may lessen the side-effects associated with either of the drugs.

Blood pressure can be controlled with monotherapy in about 50% of patients, assuming that sensible therapeutic options are adopted. It is particularly important to remember that the beta-blockers, the ACE inhibitors and possibly also the angiotensin-receptor antagonists are not particularly effective in the elderly and in African-origin patients. Diuretics and CCBs are more sensible first-line drugs for these groups.

About 40% of patients require double therapy and around 10% require triple therapy. A small minority of patients require four or even five drugs to reduce their pressure to below 160/90 mmHg. These patients should be referred to specialist clinics.

THE SECOND STEP

If optimum blood pressure control is not achieved with first-line drugs when used appropriately then another type of blood pressure drug can be added in. Some combinations are more effective than others (Figure 12.1 and Table 12.2), and some may have little additive effect, or may be potentially harmful (Table 12.3).

Table 12.2
Suggested therapeutic combinations to reduce blood pressure.

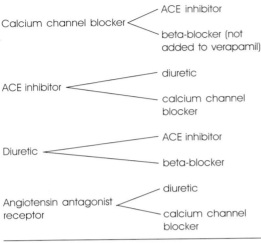

Calcium channel blocker
— ACE inhibitor
— beta-blocker (not added to verapamil)

ACE inhibitor
— diuretic
— calcium channel blocker

Diuretic
— ACE inhibitor
— beta-blocker

Angiotensin antagonist receptor
— diuretic
— calcium channel blocker

Table 12.3
Therapeutic combinations not usually recommended.

verapamil + beta-blocker
dihydropyridine + diuretic
ACE inhibitor + beta-blocker
angiotensin-antagonist receptor + ACE inhibitor
angiotensin-antagonist receptor + beta-blocker

Table 12.4
A guide to resistant blood pressure control (i.e. not controlled by two drugs).

(a) **Check compliance with lifestyle changes**
  (i)   salt restriction (check 24-hour urine)
  (ii) weight reduction where relevant
  (iii) alcohol restraint if intake excessive

(b) **Check therapeutic compliance**
  (i)   tablet counts
  (ii) monitor drug levels in blood if possible
  (iii) simplify therapeutic regime

(c) **Investigate further for underlying cause of hypertension**
  (i)   Renal arteriogram
  (ii) Urinary catecholamines
  (iii) Plasma renin/aldosterone assays

Check compliance

Enquire whether the patient is taking the prescribed drugs and whether they find the tablet regime difficult to remember. There are certain clues to non-compliance, such as the lack of fall in heart rate with a beta-blocker, or no fall in serum potassium with a thiazide diuretic. Tablet counts or discussion with relatives may produce surprises in patients who claim to be compliant with their drug regime.

Simplify the regime

Complex regimes can lead to poor compliance. It is now possible to convert all patients to a once-daily drug regime. It sometimes helps to suggest to patients that they take all their tablets when they get home in the evening, rather than first thing in the morning when they may be in a hurry.

RESISTANT HYPERTENSION

If patients have been tried on two genuinely additive drugs and blood pressure is still not controlled the outlook is poor. Table 12.4 provides a checklist of manoeuvres for such patients.

Salt restriction

Many patients may be eating large amounts of salt and this is may be an important reason for lack of response to some drugs. This can easily be checked by collecting a 24-hour urine and measuring sodium excretion, which provides a good guide to the patient's usual salt intake.

Surreptitious alcoholics

Withdrawal from a high alcohol intake can cause rises in blood pressure. Patients may stop drinking 24 hours before seeing the doctor and thus present with a falsely elevated blood pressure.

Obesity

Many hypertensive patients are overweight, and much can be achieved by referring them to a dietician who can advise on the best way of reducing weight, reducing salt intake and increasing potassium consumption with fruit and vegetables.

Check for underlying causes of hypertension

Most patients with underlying causes, such as renal artery stenosis, primary aldosteronism and phaeochromocytoma, have severe hypertension that is often resistant to therapy. It is vital that these patients are investigated to exclude renal or adrenal disease along the lines suggested in Chapter 8.

THE THIRD STEP

Patients whose blood pressure is resistant to double therapy in the combinations suggested in Table 12.2 and Figure 12.1 have a high risk of cardiovascular complications of hypertension. Such patients should be referred to specialised blood pressure clinics. Particularly, it is important to exclude an underlying cause for hypertension.

A long-acting ACE inhibitor or an angiotensin-receptor antagonist can be used combined with a long-acting calcium antagonist, with the addition of either a diuretic or a beta-blocker or both. In some patients it may be necessary to add in frusemide twice daily, or in very resistant cases the powerful diuretic metolazone, in a dose of 5 mg daily, can be used, but with care as it may cause a large increase in urine sodium and water, leading to hypotension. Metolazone does, however, cause a less rapid diuresis than frusemide and patients may be less inconvenienced.

Some clinicians recommend adding verapamil to a dihydropyridine in resistant hypertension. The addition of minoxidil may be effective in very resistant patients, but its side-effects, particularly tachycardia, hair growth and fluid retention, have limited its use.

Occasionally, a patient is encountered whose blood pressure, while never dangerously high, appears to be resistant to all treatment. It is worth checking whether the patient has only transient elevations of pressure in response to attending the clinic. If he or she rests in a quiet room for half an hour, and the blood pressure is checked by a reliably trained nurse, lower readings may be achieved. Semi-automatic blood pressure monitors may have a role, by obtaining a large number of blood pressure readings.

Twenty-four-hour ambulatory monitoring can be performed to see what level blood pressure falls to when the patient is outside the clinic environment. If such patients have normal blood pressure and absolutely no evidence of cardiac, renal or cerebral damage, and, particularly, if the ECG shows no evidence of left ventricular hypertrophy (LVH), then it may be reasonable to accept less than optimal control of clinic blood pressure. It may be, in such patients, that home blood-pressure monitoring may be a better way of controlling blood pressure.

Patients who exhibit this 'white-coat' effect cannot be regarded as normal because many of them develop genuine 'fixed' hypertension within 5 years.

MALIGNANT HYPERTENSION

All patients with the malignant phase of hypertension (i.e. those with retinal haemorrhages, exudates with or without papilloedema) should, as soon as the diagnosis has been made, be treated as a medical emergency and admitted to hospital for controlled blood pressure reduction and detailed investigation. If the blood pressure is not adequately reduced, the disease progresses rapidly to end-stage chronic renal failure requiring dialysis, or to death from cardiac failure or stroke. However, too-rapid reduction of blood pressure may be dangerous, and has been shown to cause both stroke and myocardial infarction as well as deterioration of renal function or acute renal failure. The aim, therefore, should be to lower the diastolic pressure, with the use of oral therapy, only to around 110 mmHg over a period of 24–48 hours, and to lower it to 100 mmHg after a week or two, often after

the patient has been discharged from hospital. The end the target is to reduce blood pressure to below 160/90 mmHg.

Intravenous drug therapy is only justified if there is hypertensive encephalopathy, severe hypertensive heart failure or aortic dissection.

Regimes for malignant hypertension

Beta-blockers, ACE inhibitors and CCBs will all lower blood pressure in most patients with malignant hypertension. Theoretically the ACE inhibitors have some attractions, as they directly oppose the immediate cause of high blood pressure, i.e. the high levels of angiotensin II seen in malignant-phase hypertension, However, they can cause deterioration in renal function if there is underlying, and possibly undiagnosed, renal artery stenosis, or if the patient is volume-depleted. If ACE inhibitors are used, intravenous saline should be ready in case blood pressure falls precipitously.

The CCBs are very effective in patients with malignant hypertension, but if used in a rapidly absorbed formulation they may lower blood pressure too quickly. Probably the best regime is nifedipine 10–20 mg in a tablet formulation, which has a peak effect at 1–2 hours. Many of these patients will require several drugs thereafter to control pressure. Some patients are volume-depleted and underweight, therefore it may occasionally be necessary to increase salt intake temporarily to increase body weight in order to increase perfusion of the kidneys. All these patients should be referred to a specialist unit for further investigation. Around 50% of patients with malignant hypertension have an underlying cause such as a phaeochromocytoma, renal artery stenosis or parenchymal renal diseases. Primary aldosteronism may rarely present with malig-nant-phase hypertension.

HYPERTENSIVE EMERGENCIES

Many antihypertensive drugs can be given intravenously or intramuscularly and lower blood pressure very rapidly. They were, and in some cases continue to be, used far too widely in hospital practice. The danger of precipitating a stroke or heart attack outweighs any benefit that may be gained from rapid reduction of blood pressure. However, in patients with hypertensive encephalopathy, gross left ventricular failure directly due to the severe hypertension, or dissecting aortic aneurysm, intravenous treatment is mandatory.

All such patients should be admitted to an intensive care unit, and an intra-arterial line should be inserted to measure blood pressure directly and continuously.

Diazoxide

This drug has been widely used as a parenteral agent and, some years ago, it was recommended to be given rapidly as an intravenous bolus of 300 mg. This produced an immediate and precipitous fall in blood pressure of 30–40% within 2–3 minutes, and serious complications were described. A safer way of giving diazoxide is either by infusion or in 50 mg intravenous injections given slowly and not repeated for at least 10 minutes. This will give a gradual reduc-tion in blood pressure over 30 minutes to 2 hours to the desired level, thereby avoiding any precipitous falls.

Labetalol

Labetalol is a combined alpha-beta-blocker but predominantly has alpha-blocking activities when given intravenously. It will lower blood pressure rapidly when given as an infusion. This regime is favoured by obstetricians when managing patients with severe eclampsia.

Nitroprusside

This is a potent vasodilator that invariably lowers blood pressure when given by intra-venous infusion. The fall in blood pressure can be controlled by the rate of infusion. However, it must be given under very close supervision as severe hypotension can easily occur. It should be reserved for use in inten-sive care units or by anaesthetists. As well as causing the expected side-effects of any arteriolar vasodilator, i.e. flushing and postu-ral hypotension, nitroprusside is metabolised to cyanide and thiacyanate. This is not impor-tant during short-term infusion, but toxicity can develop if the drug is given over several days, particularly when there is renal failure.

New solutions need to be made up every 4 hours and must be covered by light-proof paper to prevent photodeactivation. The usual starting dose is 0.5 µg/kg per minute to a maximum of 8 µg/kg per minute. Blood pressure should be measured extremely carefully and the amount of nitroprusside should be carefully monitored.

Hydralazine

Hydralazine can be given either intravenously or intramuscularly and was once widely used, but is now only used by obstetricians. The normal dose is 10–40 mg injected slowly. In most situations where it is used, oral hydralazine would be just as effective.

Oral therapy

For patients able to take drugs by mouth, most antihypertensive drugs given orally act rapidly. For instance, nifedipine given in a 10 mg capsule will cause blood pressure to fall within 10–15 minutes. The ACE inhibitor, captopril, when taken orally will lower blood pressure within 30 minutes. Oral beta-blockers, with or without hydralazine, reduce blood pressure over a period of 2–3 hours.

FURTHER READING

Carruthers SG, Larochelle P, Haynes RB, *et al.* Report of the Canadian Hypertension Society Consensus Conference — 1 Introduction. *Canad Med Ass J* 1993; **149**: 289–93.

Guidelines Sub-Committee. 1993 Guidelines for the management of mild hypertension: memorandum for a World Heath Organisation/International Hypertension Society. *J Hypertens* 1993; **11**: 905–18.

Gibbs CR, Kong KL, Churchill D, *et al.* The management of hypertensive crisis. *Care Critic III* 1996; **12**: 172–6.

Jackson R, Barham P, Bills T, *et al.* Management of raised blood pressure in New Zealand: a discussion document. *Br Med J* 1993; **307**: 107–10.

Sever PS, Beevers DG, Bulpitt CJ, *et al.* Management guidelines in essential hypertension: report of the second working party of the British Hypertension Society. *Br Med J* 1993; **306**: 983–7.

13

HYPERTENSION IN PRIMARY MEDICAL CARE

BACKGROUND

Other chapters in this book have dealt with the epidemiology, aetiology, investigation and treatment of high blood pressure. The next question is, who actually should deliver this potentially life-saving treatment? There is evidence that the quality and efficiency of blood pressure reduction on a long-term basis is a more potent predictor of a patient's life expectancy than the severity of the hypertension in the first place. Regrettably, practically every population survey in the UK, the USA and elsewhere has reported a depressing state of underdiagnosis, undertreatment and inadequate follow-up of hypertensive patients. The 'rule of halves' described in Chapter 1 means that less than 15% of all hypertensive patients are receiving adequate clinical care. The need for improvement in the detection and management of hypertension ranks with the abolition of cigarette smoking as a major public health concern in developed countries. In the developing countries, this new epidemic is just around the corner, unless steps are actively taken to avoid it.

As most hypertensive people have only mildly elevated blood pressures, and complain of no symptoms, they are not likely to present to hospital specialists. The hospital-based services are, therefore, in no position to influence the problem of the rule of halves. The detection and management of millions of hypertensive people (up to 20% of the adult population) must therefore be the responsibility of the doctors and nurses in the primary health care system. This is in line with a trend for general practitioners (GPs) to undertake an increased and more systematic role in the management of other chronic conditions including hyperlipidaemia, diabetes mellitus, asthma and arthritis.

PRIMARY HEALTH CARE

The system for the delivery of primary health care varies from country to country. In some parts of the world, there is no systematic or established system for primary and preventive medical care, whereas a recognised speciality known as family medicine, or general practice, has been in place in some countries for many years. It is within the context of the primary health care team that most hypertensive patients should be managed, so each nation has to adapt its health care resources to take on the challenge of managing millions of hypertensive patients. The pay-off is the prevention of deaths due to heart attack and stroke.

General practice

In the UK, every citizen has a named GP who is responsible for the immediate care of a specified number of patients on his or her list. With the exception of accidents and emergencies, the individual patient must go to the GP as the first medical contact, and will only be referred to a specialist if the GP considers it necessary. This system was established in 1948 and has undergone radical changes since that time, with a steady improvement in standards. General practice is now recognised as a speciality in its own right, with its own organised system of postgraduate training and qualifications. In addition, most GPs have now pooled their resources, and work in modern, purpose-built, community-based health centres or medical centres. With this trend towards group practices, many individual GPs have tended to take up special interests, providing care for particular conditions for their whole group practice. There is increasing skill and expertise amongst the doctors in the primary health care system and this trend is to be encouraged.

Nurse practitioners

Perhaps the most significant development in the field of primary health care has been the establishment of the system of practice nurses. In many primary health care teams, the number of nurses has equalled the number of doctors. There is now increasing evidence that appropriately trained nurses can take on the management of many chronic diseases such as diabetes mellitus, asthma and, of course, hypertension. In general, student nurse training has in the past tended to be geared mainly towards the care of acutely sick patients in hospital. Particular efforts are now necessary to organise suitable training schemes to enable nurses to fulfil an increasingly important role in the field of hypertension care. Nurses are ideally suited for counselling their patients on lifestyle changes, which have been shown to aid in the prevention as well as in the treatment of all grades of hypertension. In addition, they have a major role to play in managing the other important risk factors for coronary heart disease.

Nurses Hypertension Associations have now been established both in the UK and Australia in order to disseminate information and encourage research. Perhaps it is a sign of the times that in 1997, Professor Martha Hill, a hypertension nurse specialist, was elected as president of the American Heart Association.

Health maintenance organisations

There is an increasing trend in the USA for the development of a system of primary health care where the detection and management of chronic diseases and, where possible, their prevention is the main priority. These initiatives are carried out by Health Maintenance Organisations (HMOs) in a system not unlike that which exists in the UK. The speciality of family medicine is expanding in the USA; it differs from the system in the UK in many respects but the objectives are similar. Private insurance schemes and occupational health programmes are also now intimately involved in primary prevention in the USA.

Primary health care in developing countries

Hypertension is emerging as a major cause of premature death in developing countries. With urbanisation, blood pressures rise sharply, and hypertension is now a common condition, particularly in the economically active segment of the population. This presents the health care systems of developing countries with a new problem, no less devastating than the epidemics of infectious disease and the problems of malnutrition. There is a need, therefore, to establish a system to deliver efficient primary health care in order to tackle the new epidemics of hypertension, diabetes mellitus, coronary heart disease and strokes. Each individual developing country must find its own solutions, but with the relatively small numbers of qualified doctors it is likely that, as in the developed countries, there is an increasing role for various forms of paramedical staff, nurse practitioners and 'bare-foot doctors'. Again, training programmes are necessary in the skills of detection and management of hypertension as well as its prevention, particularly with dietary and lifestyle advice.

SCREENING FOR HYPERTENSION

The symptomless nature of the earlier stages of hypertension means that some sort of screening initiative is necessary if hypertensive patients are to be detected and heart attacks and strokes prevented. The exact method to be employed depends on the primary health care system in individual countries. Most of the systems discussed below are relevant to the health care system in developed countries, but the basic principals are relevant for all nations.

Selective screening

A very strong case has been made for the selective screening of people who are at particular risk of developing the vascular complications of hypertension.

Family history

It should be the responsibility of patients as well as doctors to seek out symptomless relatives of those people who have been diagnosed as having hypertension or its complications, particularly heart attack and stroke. Many of these relatives will have raised blood pressure themselves and may benefit from antihypertensive treatment. Similarly, such patients should be screened to detect hyperlipidaemia. These high-risk individuals need active counselling if they are to avoid the same fate as their unhealthy family members.

Previous complications

Patients who have already suffered a vascular complication of hypertension have a very high risk of recurrence. Second strokes can be prevented if blood pressure is controlled on a long-term basis. People who have already sustained a myocardial infarct need very active care. There is abundant evidence that heart attack recurrence can be reduced with active drug treatment using beta-blockers or verapamil, even if the patient is normotensive. Furthermore, there is now evidence that ACE inhibition is beneficial in post-infarct patients with poor ventricular systolic function. Similarly, the management of hyperlipidaemia even at this late stage is definitely beneficial, and smoking cessation is still worthwhile. Long-term low-dose aspirin is of proven benefit in survivors of heart attack.

Diabetes mellitus

There is increasing awareness that in diabetic patients, the height of the blood pressure is often more important than the severity of the glucose intolerance. All diabetics should have regular blood pressure checks (Chapter 14).

Systemic diseases

The presence of hypertension substantially worsens the prognosis in a great many unrelated medical conditions, and all patients with rheumatoid arthritis and collagen vascular diseases, endocrine abnormalities and renal diseases need regular screening for hypertension (see Chapter 14).

Pregnancy

Another high risk group is pregnant women, where hypertension remains an important cause of perinatal and maternal morbidity and mortality. Here, the efficient detection and management of high blood pressure is already an integral part of good routine obstetric care (see Chapter 16). The rest of

the medical profession have a lot to learn from this.

Mass screening

The so-called 'well population screening' of fit populations is an emotive issue. Screening alone is not enough; there must also be efficient follow-up of abnormalities detected. Mass screening using mobile screening units is an efficient means of recruiting patients for clinical trials, but obviously if this is only a one-off exercise, it cannot solve an ongoing long-term problem.

Occupational screening

Screening of employees clearly has its place, but this is available to only a minority of the population, mainly men who are employed in large firms or industries. There are also problems of confidentiality of clinical information, and usually industrial medical officers do not organise follow-up or drug treatment of chronic medical conditions. However, occupational health teams, particularly with the aid of nurses, can provide a supportive role in the management of hypertension in their work force.

Medical insurance companies

Private medical insurance in the UK has not addressed the problem of the early detection and management of cardiovascular risk factors, even though this may prove cost-effective. In the USA and elsewhere, the insurance industry has developed various forms of screening programmes and thus made an important contribution to the detection and management of hypertension and other coronary risk factors.

Casual screening

The provision of blood pressure measurement equipment and staff in supermarkets, department stores and public places can make only a small impact without follow-up and treatment. There is evidence that casual screening programmes such as these tend to attract hypertensive patients who are already diagnosed; people whose pressures have never been measured tend to ignore them. Increased public health education may alter this tendency, but the system is certainly not ideal at present.

Screening in the primary health care system

In developed countries, more than 75% of the adult population see a doctor for some reason at least once over a period of 3 years, and this almost invariably occurs in the context of primary health care. The methods to be used to screen for hypertension in primary care must vary from country to country, but the system described below has the potential to detect almost all cases of hypertension and is adaptable for differing health care delivery systems.

In an ideal world, every person from childhood upwards would have his or her blood pressure measured as a routine procedure. Screening people below the age of about 20 would, however, yield relatively few hypertensive cases. Furthermore, the benefits of screening and intervention in

Table 13.1

Estimated number of patients who are registered with an average British general practice who have a single casual blood pressure of 160/95 mmHg or more. Figures in brackets denote the percentage of people in that age band with hypertension.

Age	Men	Women
0-19	7 (2%)	4 (1%)
20-39	25 (7%)	8 (3%)
40-59	70 (25%)	52 (18%)
60-79	66 (35%)	93 (37%)
80+	10 (50%)	26 (50%)
Total	178	183

very mild hypertension in childhood and adolescence are unknown.

Screening all people over the age of 80 would produce a very large number of abnormalities, but this would be in a group of patients in whom the benefits of treating mild hypertension are less certain.

A reasonable compromise is for case detection programmes to be instituted for everyone between the ages of 20 and 80. This represents about 1500 examinees in an average general practice in the UK, where there are about 2000 people on each GP's list. Of those examinees, about 20% (300 people) would have blood pressures above 160/95 mmHg (Table 13.1). All such individuals would need rechecking and, in many, blood pressures will fall. Only if blood pressures remain above this level after rechecking on four occasions should drug therapy be considered. Very severe hypertension is rare in general practice but clearly, when it is present, more urgent action is necessary.

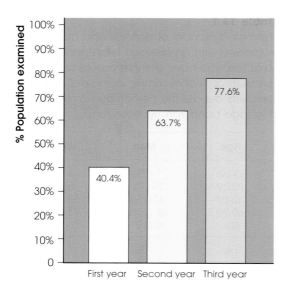

Figure 13.1
Proportion of eligible population examined by opportunistic screening in general practice in Scotland.

Opportunistic screening

This system, which has been employed in many countries, relies on the observation that most people seek a medical consultation at least once in 3 years. This represents an ideal time to arrange for screening for hypertension as well as other symptomless medical conditions. In women, cervical cytology and breast examination can be organised at the same time.

The term 'opportunistic screening' implies that the doctor takes the opportunity provided by the patient's attendance to do routine checks. By this method, 75–80% of the population can be screened with no special efforts, appointments or clinics. Suitably trained nurses are probably the best people to conduct these routine tests and to discuss with the patients their lifestyles, cooking habits and perceived health problems. The system has proved workable: it can be ongoing and appropriate follow-up is easy to arrange (Fig. 13.1).

Appointments for eligible examinees

A faster way is to arrange appointments for all patients to have a routine blood pressure check, which will require extra paperwork and time spent on documentation, postage and screening clinics. However, it can achieve a complete screen over a period of a few months and is useful as a system to initiate a well-population screening service and can take place at the same time as opportunistic screening.

Screening of newly eligible patients

Once the backlog of previously unscreened patients has been examined, it is important to continue the programme to include individuals who become eligible for screening over the ensuing years. For this purpose, the doctor should ideally have an age/sex register of the patients on the practice list. Patients reaching the age of 20 can thus be summoned for screening. One GP in England sends his patients a birthday card together with an appointment for a blood pressure and general health check.

Moving house

In the UK, when an individual moves to live in a new area, they will usually visit the local health centre and join the list of that practice. In time, their NHS medical records will be sent to their new doctor. If the

Figure 13.2
A patient-held BP record card.

```
┌─────────────────────────────────────────────┐
│  HYPERTENSION COOPERATION CARD                │
│                                               │
│  Name: Thomas Smith    DOB 27/9/33            │
│  Address: 47 Anstrother steet                 │
│  Westchester   Loamshire                      │
│  ............ Post Code W27 9BU               │
│                                               │
│  General Practitioner: Dr Antrobus            │
│                                               │
│  Date diagnosed hypertensive 16/2/94          │
│  Cigarette smoking  No /(Yes) Quantity 20/d   │
│  Advice:                                      │
│  (1) avoid being overweight                   │
│  (2) moderate alcohol consumption             │
│  (3) restrict salt intake                     │
│  (4) show this card to all doctors and nurses who look │
│      after you                                │
│  (5) always bring your tablets when consulting your │
│      doctor or nurse                          │
│  (6) don't stop taking tablets unless advised to by your │
│      doctor or nurse                          │
│  (7) your target blood pressure is below      │
│      160/90mmHg                               │
└─────────────────────────────────────────────┘
```

(a)

DATE	16/2/94	19/3/94	17/5/94	21/7/94	19/6/94	17/11/94	12/1/95	6/5/95	19/8/95	27/11/95
B.P.1	172/106	170/102	168/100	152/92	156/94	154/90	138/84	136/82	132/84	134/82
PULSE	98	82								
B.P. 2	168/98	168/98	172/98	148/90	152/92	152/94	134/80	132/78	135/83	128/80
URINE	NAD	✓								
WEIGHT kg st lbs	84.2	84.0	82.1	81.6	82.0	82.2	84.0	82.4	81.0	80.2
DRUG 1 Bendroflvazide	✓	✓	start 2.5mg	2.5m	stop	✓	✓	✓	✓	✓
DRUG 2 Lisinopril	✓	✓	✓		start 10mg	increase 20mg	20mg	20m	20m	20m
DRUG 3	✓	✓	✓	✓	✓	✓	✓	✓	✓	✓
DRUG 4	✓	✓	✓	✓	✓	✓	✓	✓	✓	✓
DRUG 5	✓	✓	✓	✓	✓	✓	✓	✓	✓	✓
DRUG 6 SIMVASTATIN	✓	✓	✓	✓	✓	✓	start 10mg	✓	increase 20mg	20
SERUM UREA	6.2	✓	✓	✓	✓	6.0	✓	✓	✓	✓
SERUM CHOLESTEROL	7.6	✓	✓	✓	✓	7.4	✓	6.2	6.7	5.5
OTHER INVESTIGATIONS	No	✓	✓	✓	✓	✓	✓	✓	✓	✓
NEXT VISIT	1/12	2/12	2/12	3/12	1/12	2/12	3/12	3/12	3/12	2/12
DOCTOR's SIGNATURE	RA	AO	RA	RA	RA	RA	RA	RA	RA	AO

(b)

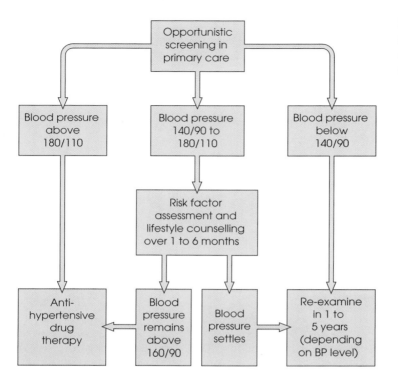

Figure 13.3
Suggested action in primary care during opportunistic screening programmes.

patient has not undergone appropriate routine checks with their previous GP, or if an abnormality was detected, the new primary health care team should arrange for routine checking as described above.

Medical records

Efficient medical records are mandatory if patients are to receive good medical care. The advent of 'user-friendly' computerised record systems can greatly help in the detection, assessment and follow-up of hypertensive patients.

The creation of age/sex registers of all patients attached to an individual health centre and from this the creation of diagnostic lists

or disease registers can greatly help in the management of patients and can be useful in creating an audit system.

However, even if a computerised system is not available, primary health care can be delivered with equal efficiency. In the UK, the GP records system (the Lloyd George Envelope) is adaptable and can be used to draw attention visually to the records of patients requiring screening or, following screening, needing special care.

Any type of sticker, or protruding section of an inserted card, renders individual patient's records readily identifiable. These can be used to draw attention to important diagnoses, not only of hypertension, and to identify patients due for blood pressure checking. The system has been used in many practices and it is simple, cheap and effective.

The principle described here can be adapted for use in any health care system anywhere, so it is relevant to all countries. In view of the fact that computerised systems can occasionally break down, some sort of manual back-up system is probably desirable anyway.

Patient-held records

With increasingly mobile communities, it is sometimes useful for patients to have a copy of their medical records, in which blood pressure and the other cardiovascular risk factors can be recorded and follow-up data added (Fig. 13.2). This system can also be used to aid in the shared care of hypertensive patients who attend a hospital-based blood pressure clinic as well as seeing their GP. There is evidence that when patients are fully informed about their blood pressure and have an accurate list of the drugs they are meant to be taking, then compliance with medical advice is improved.

Blood pressure screening and subsequent action

When blood pressure is measured at first screening, there are three possible outcomes, i.e. triage (Fig. 13.3). The pressure may be entirely normal (diastolic pressure below 90 mmHg and systolic blood pressure below 140 mmHg) so no action is necessary for some years. However, counselling on the avoidance of hypertension and cardiovascular disease may be worthwhile. The second possibility is that the pressure is found to be so high (diastolic BP of 110 mmHg or more, systolic BP 180 mmHg or more) that action is necessary more or less immediately. The large intermediate group represents patients who have mildly elevated blood pressures (140/90 to 180/110), many of which will settle on rechecking. This group needs very careful assessment in order to avoid over-treatment.

Mild hypertension

The guidelines of the United States Joint National Committee (JNC-VI) and the British Hypertension Society strongly advocate the careful assessment of mild hypertensive patients before drug therapy is initiated.

There is evidence that whilst blood pressures fall on rechecking, they tend to level out after the fourth visit. These follow-up visits, best organised by a primary health care nurse, can also be used as an opportunity to provide the patient with counselling about important dietary changes that may be necessary, together, where relevant, with advice on smoking cessation and alcohol moderation. Only if the diastolic blood pressure remains above 90 mmHg or the systolic pressure remains above 160 mmHg at the fourth visit, should antihypertensive drugs be considered.

The schemes for reducing blood pressure are dealt with in detail in Chapter 12. The majority of hypertensive patients can be managed very adequately in primary care and in only a minority will blood pressure remain uncontrolled.

Investigations in general practice

The methods for investigating hypertensive patients are discussed in detail in Chapters

7 and 8. In general practice, all patients who require drug therapy should undergo routine first-line investigations. Urine testing is mandatory, and a single non-fasting blood test should be taken for estimation of blood glucose and serum levels of cholesterol (including HDL), urea, creatinine, sodium, potassium, calcium, urate and gamma glutamyl transferase. In addition, all patients should have a simple 12 lead ECG. Chest X-rays are not particularly useful unless the radiologist reports the cardiothoracic ratio (CTR).

Audit

The marked improvements in medical records that have taken place over the last 10 years with the increased availability of computers now provide the clinician with an opportunity to conduct clinical audit. Audit should ideally be ongoing, and the lessons learnt should lead to feedback in order to modify clinical practice. All clinicians should, therefore, establish a system to investigate how effective they have been in screening their patients for hypertension and to ensure that all cases have undergone the appropriate investigations. Furthermore, it is important to check that all hypertensive patients have their blood pressures controlled with diastolic pressures below 90 mmHg and all systolic pressures below 160 mmHg. When audit demonstrates that this is not being achieved, clinical practice should be modified and, where relevant, made more efficient.

Audit, or clinical enquiry, is now an integral part of good medical care and, of course, it also has a major pay-off in the generation of research data. In many countries, major randomised controlled drug trials of hypertensive treatment have been conducted in general practice. Sadly, however, apart from these, the impact of primary care on research into the epidemiology and treatment of hypertension has been disappointing. There is a great potential with the use of audit for an expansion of GP input into research on the nature of hypertension and its response to treatment.

REFERRAL FOR SPECIALIST ADVICE

About 10% of hypertensive patients need referral for specialist advice. These include those cases where first-line investigations suggest the presence of some underlying cause for the raised blood pressure and cases where there is evidence of end-organ damage, e.g. proteinuria, renal failure or angina, which requires detailed hospital-based investigation. In addition, mild hypertensive patients under the age of 40 should probably be referred in order to undergo detailed investigations, even if the first-line tests are unhelpful. Finally, if blood pressure remains uncontrolled, despite adequate non-pharmacological and pharmacological therapy, then specialist referral is necessary.

CONCLUSIONS

There is abundant evidence that most hypertensive patients are not receiving adequate medical care. Only a minority have their pressure reduced to below 160/90 mmHg. If, as in the USA, we reduce the target pressure to 140/90 mmHg then the figures are even more depressing. It is also clear from this chapter that the primary health care team has the facilities and the staff to solve the problem of undertreatment. If this is so, where are things going wrong? Lack of information, lack of motivation and a disorganised follow-up system could be some of the reasons.

We firmly believe that the responsibility for the control of blood pressure rests squarely in general practice. It follows that the responsibility for the failure to control blood pressure also rests squarely in general practice. Otherwise some might say that hypertension is too important to be left to GPs.

The control of blood pressure can bring about a 40% reduction in strokes and a 20–30% reduction in heart attacks in hypertensive patients. This being so, when these events do occur, the clinician should question, within the context of medical audit, whether the management of the individual patient has been adequate.

FURTHER READING

Barber JH, Beevers DG, Fife R, *et al*. Blood pressure screening and supervision in general practice. *Br Med J* 1979; **I**: 843–6.

Coope JR. ABC of blood pressure management: management in general practice. *Br Med J* 1981; **282**: 1380–2.

Coops JR, Warrender TS. Randomised trial of treatment of hypertension in elderly patients in primary care. *Br Med J* 1986; **293**: 1145–51.

Curzio JL, Beevers M. The role of nurses in hypertension care and research. *J Hum Hypertens* 1997; **11**: 541–50.

Fullard E, Fowler G, Gray M. Facilitating prevention in primary care. *Br Med J* 1984; **289**: 1585–7.

Joint National Committee on Detection, Evaluation and Treatment of High Blood Pressure. The Sixth Report of the Joint National Committee on Prevention, Detection, Evaluation and Treatment of High Blood Pressure (JNC VI). *Arch Intern Med* 1997; **157**: 2413–46.

Juncosa S, Jones RB, McGhee SM. Appropriateness of hospital referral for hypertension. *Br Med J* 1990; **300**: 646–8.

Kurj KH, Haines AP. Detection and management of hypertension in general practice in north-west London. *Br Med J* 1984; **288**: 903–5.

Sever P, Beevers DG, Bulpitt CJ, *et al*. Management guidelines in essential hypertension: report of the second working party of the British Hypertension Society. *Br Med J* 1993; **306**: 983–7.

Whitfield M, Hughes A. Hypertension management in general practice. *J R Soc Med* 1997; **90**: 12–15.

4

Section Four

14

HYPERTENSION WITH OTHER DISEASES

BACKGROUND

No two hypertensive patients are alike, and very few of them resemble those highly selected cases included in the long-term randomised trials discussed in Chapter 9. In reality, patients differ in the severity of their hypertension, the frequency of pre-existing vascular complications and the presence of concomitant medical conditions which themselves substantially influence clinical management. Trial participants tend to be relatively low-risk individuals who are fit enough and have sufficient motivation to enter long-term studies. Clinical practice is rather different. In this chapter, we discuss the impact of other diagnoses on the investigation and management of hypertension. First, we cover the presence of pre-existing vascular diseases that may in part be the consequence of raised blood pressure; then we discuss the importance of related vascular risk factors, like diabetes mellitus and plasma lipid levels, and their impact on antihypertensive therapy. Finally we discuss the presence of important but unrelated medical conditions.

There are practically no medical specialities where the presence of hypertension does not substantially influence the outlook, and all specialists need to be aware of the impact of hypertension on their clinical decision making. Furthermore, the frequency and importance of other medical conditions increases with advancing age as does the prevalence of hypertension itself.

HYPERTENSION AND ITS VASCULAR COMPLICATIONS

Hypertension and heart disease

As high blood pressure is an important risk factor for coronary heart disease, it is hardly surprising that many patients have cardiac damage, particularly as they get older.

Patients may have other causes for heart disease at the same time, including rheumatic heart disease, cor pulmonale or a cardiomyopathy. Beta-blockers, ACE inhibitors and more recently angiotensin-receptor antagonists are themselves used in the treatment of some forms of heart disease in patients with normal blood pressure as well as in hypertensive patients.

Angina pectoris

Many hypertensive patients have anginal pain. This is only partly related to an increased tendency to develop coronary atheroma. Hypertensive patients with marked LVH may develop lateral ST-T changes in leads V4 to V6 of their ECG due to relative ischaemia (sometimes called 'strain') where the cardiac enlargement is not accompanied by an appropriate increase in vascular supply. Many hypertensive patients with severe or unstable angina are found on coronary angiography to have relatively little coronary artery narrowing.

The effective lowering of blood pressure by any class of antihypertensive drug does reduce the severity and frequency of angina pectoris. However, beta-blockers and calcium-channel blockers have specific anti-anginal properties, in addition to their antihypertensive effects. Beta-blockers remain the first choice but where these are ineffective, or contraindicated, the calcium-channel blockers (nifedipine or amlodipine) are reasonable second-line drugs and can be combined with a beta-blocker. Both verapamil and diltiazem are also effective. If angina still persists, then long-acting oral nitrates (e.g. isosorbide mononitrate) should be added. All patients with angina should be assessed carefully, usually with an exercise ECG. If blood pressure is well controlled and angina persists, coronary surgery or angioplasty should be considered. It is worth remembering that an exercise ECG may be difficult to interpret if there is underlying LVH with strain, as the ST segments may be depressed even at rest. In such cases, it may be better to do a radionuclide (e.g. thallium) scan or proceed directly to angiography.

Myocardial infarction

All patients, and thus all hypertensive patients, who sustain a heart attack should be given a beta-blocker in addition to low-dose aspirin unless there are contraindications. Both of these have been shown to reduce the reinfarction rate over the ensuing years. One report demonstrated that if beta-blockers are contraindicated, then a similar degree of secondary prevention can be achieved with verapamil. ACE inhibitors are also beneficial in post-infarction patients, particularly if they have poor left ventricular systolic function; not only is clinical cardiac failure prevented but there appears also to be a lower rate of reinfarction.

During 1995 a series of papers raised anxieties about the use of the calcium-channel blockers. Whilst these have now been allayed by the publication of the results of the SYST-EUR trial in 1997, one contraindication does remain. In post-infarct patients and those with unstable angina the short-acting (capsule or tablet) formulations of nifedipine should not be used. We believe that they should not be used in any patients anyway. With their sudden onset and rapid elimination they cause catecholamine surges, which may provoke lethal arrhythmias.

The above comments are relevant to all patients following a heart attack whether or not they are also hypertensive. If the patient is hypertensive, the clinician should be aware of some other factors that influence diagnosis and management.

First, the incidence of silent or symptom-less myocardial infarction is greater in hypertensive patients compared with normotensive patients and the prognosis for hypertensives following a heart attack is bad.

Second, following myocardial infarction, blood pressure may fall so that the diagnosis of hypertension may be missed. Frequently, at follow-up blood pressures rise again. The clinician must be aware, therefore, that a patient whose pressures were normal or even low whilst in the coronary

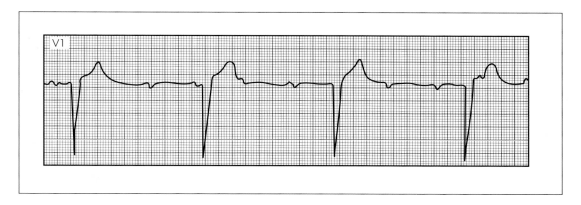

Figure 14.1
ECG showing complete heartblock.

care unit may have hypertension that may reappear after recovery.

A third and important point is that the thiazide diuretics when used in the treatment of hypertension may cause hypokalaemia and that heart attack patients with low serum potassium levels have a higher risk of arrhythmias and sudden death. A measurement of serum potassium at first presentation is mandatory in all heart attack patients, along with an assay of the cardiac enzymes and serum lipid levels.

On long-term follow-up of hypertensive patients, blood pressure must be controlled, and attention should be paid to concomitant risk factors such as cigarette smoking, diabetes mellitus and the height of the serum cholesterol concentration. The Scandinavian Simvastatin Survival Study (SSSS) clearly showed that lives were saved if an HMG CoA reductase inhibitor (a statin) was prescribed for post-infarct patients with serum cholesterol levels above 5.2 mmol/l. Almost all hypertensive patients are obese

and have cholesterol levels above this threshold. A useful rule of thumb is that almost all hypertensive patients who have had a heart attack and those with angina should be treated with simvastatin or a related compound.

Arrhythmias

The presence of any form of heart block is an absolute contraindication to beta-blockade or verapamil therapy (Fig. 14.1). The use of these two drugs together is particularly dangerous in post-infarction patients. The diagnosis of atrial fibrillation (AF) should raise the possibility of this being due to, or aggravated by, other medical conditions like hyperthyroidism or alcohol abuse, particularly if the fibrillation is resistant to digoxin. AF can, on rare occasions, be due to raised blood pressure alone. It is now known that most patients with AF should be anticoagulated with

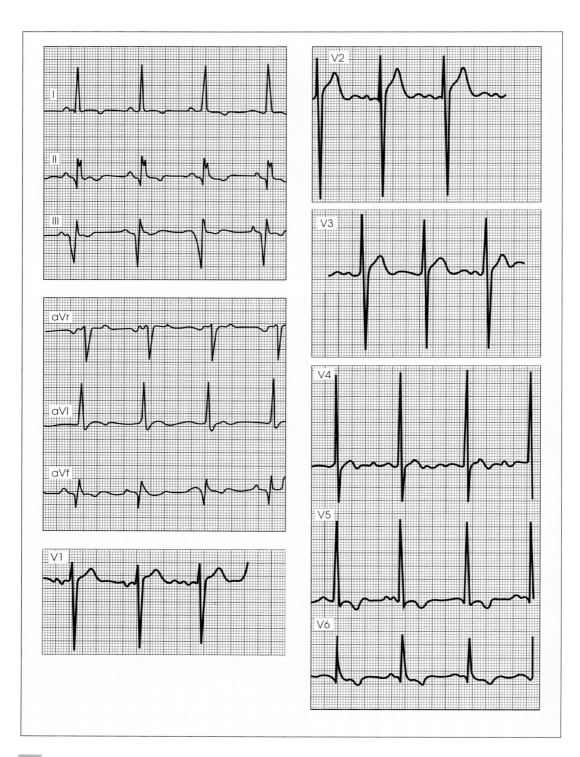

warfarin, as even in the absence of mitral valve disease, there is an increased risk of cerebral embolism. Most patients with recent onset AF should be returned to sinus rhythm if possible by chemical or electrical cardioversion.

Heart failure

ACE inhibitors and angiotensin-receptor antagonists have both been shown convincingly to prolong life in patients with heart failure. The heart failure may be due to coronary heart disease or to hypertension alone (Fig. 14.2). Other causes of heart failure including alcoholic cardiomyopathy should be considered in hypertensive patients. Beta-blockers and verapamil are contraindicated, although there is some evidence that carvedilol may be beneficial in some patients with heart failure.

Whilst ACE inhibitors or angiotensin-receptor antagonists are indicated in practically all patients with heart failure, they should be introduced with great caution. These patients may have extensive atheromatous disease and there may be concomitant but undiagnosed atheromatous renal artery stenosis. Furthermore, patients with heart failure may also be receiving treatment with frusemide and may have some intravascular volume depletion. In both these circumstances, the introduction of a drug that blocks the renin–angiotensin system may cause profound hypotension and a deterioration in renal function. It is best to start with the short-acting ACE inhibitor

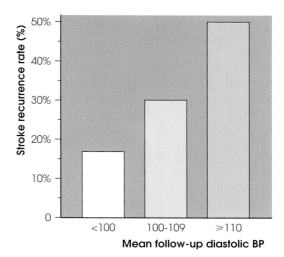

Figure 14.3

Stroke recurrence rates in relation to control of blood pressure in moderate to severe hypertension.

Figure 14.2

ECG taken from a hypertensive patient with uncontrolled severe hypertension that shows gross LVH on an old inferior myocardial infarction.

captopril in a test dose of 6.25 mg, and to monitor the blood pressure at 15 minute intervals for 3 hours. Serum creatinine levels should be rechecked after 24 hours and 5 days. On a long-term basis, a longer-acting, ACE inhibitor should be prescribed in the full dose (eg lisinopril 20 mg daily) even if the blood pressure is controlled with lower doses.

If ACE inhibitors cannot be used due to side-effects, we feel it is justifiable to use an angiotensin-receptor antagonist, even though this class of drug is not yet licensed for heart failure. This is because a reliable study (the ELITE trial) demonstrated in 1997 that losartan was as good as, or possibly even better than, captopril in the treatment of heart failure in the elderly.

The use of hydralazine in combination with a nitrate has also been shown to save lives in heart failure, but the benefits were less marked than with ACE inhibitors or losartan. However, the combination of hydralazine and nitrates may be the most effective in Afro-Caribbean patients with heart failure.

Acute and very severe heart failure may be due to very severe hypertension alone. If the blood pressure is lowered, the heart failure may improve. Sodium nitroprusside by infusion in a dose of 0.02–0.5 mg/minute can provide very accurate minute to minute control of blood pressure, whilst avoiding precipitate and dangerous episodes of hypotension. In less severe cases, oral nifedipine in tablet (not capsule) form may be used (see Chapter 12).

Hypertension and stroke

Whilst strokes are four times less common than heart attacks in middle-aged hypertensives patients, the incidence is roughly equal in the elderly. Antihypertensive treatment is particularly effective in preventing strokes in all age groups. If a hypertensive patient does sustain a stroke, then the clinician should investigate 'what went wrong?' and in some cases, medical negligence should be considered.

Stroke recurrence

In a hypertensive patient who has sustained a stroke, the mechanism is much more likely to be a cerebral infarction than cerebral haemorrhage. A CT or MRI scan to confirm the diagnosis and differentiate between infarction and haemorrhage is mandatory in order to decide whether aspirin therapy or even early thrombolysis should be prescribed.

Immediate or rapid blood pressure reduction is dangerous. Following a stroke, cerebral autoregulation is broken down so that falls in blood pressure directly cause falls in cerebral perfusion.

There remains a degree of uncertainty about the optimum management of hypertension in stroke survivors. It is our policy to continue with existing antihypertensive therapy, if possible using oral agents. In all patients we would only recommend initiating new therapies in the acute stage if the systolic pressure consistently exceeds 180 mmHg and the diastolic pressure consistently exceeds 110 mmHg. Under these circumstances we would prescribe oral atenolol starting on a dose of 25 mg or nifedipine in tablet form starting with 10 mg daily. Our aim would be to reduce the pressure to no lower than 160/100 mmHg in the first 24 hours.

In stroke survivors, on a long-term basis the adequate control of moderate to severe hypertension is associated with a major reduction in the frequency of stroke recurrence (Fig. 14.3). There is also a close relationship between strokes and cigarette smoking and heavy alcohol consumption, so, where appropriate, sympathetic constructive counselling is necessary. Although no dedicated trial has investigated the value of lipid lowering in stroke survivors, we would prescribe this if the serum cholesterol is greater than 5.0 mmol/l. It is interesting that in the SSSS trial of lipid lowering in heart attack patients, there was also a statistically significant reduction in strokes in patients receiving the active drug, when compared with the placebo group.

Subarachnoid haemorrhage

There is a close association between hypertension and subarachnoid haemorrhage. Cigarette smoking is also a major risk factor.

All patients need careful assessment to exclude the diagnosis of underlying autosomal dominant polycystic kidney disease (PKD). A detailed family history may reveal relatives with renal failure, stroke or subarachnoid haemorrhage. The diagnosis of PKD is best made non-invasively with a renal ultrasound scan.

Once the diagnosis of subarachnoid haemorrhage is confirmed, either by CT scan or lumbar puncture, it is now known to be helpful to prescribe the calcium-channel blocker, nimodipine, in order to reduce or prevent spasm of the surrounding cerebral vessels. If the blood pressure remains high, a beta-blocker should be added in. If a berry aneurysm is found, neurosurgical treatment is mandatory. On a long-term basis, careful control of blood pressure is very important to prevent recurrence.

Peripheral vascular disease

Peripheral vascular disease is closely related to blood pressure, serum cholesterol levels and cigarette smoking. There is, as yet, little evidence from clinical trials that any drug therapy favourably influences the outcome, and some antihypertensive drugs have side-effects that make things worse (e.g. thiazides may further raise cholesterol and beta-blockers cause cold extremities and may worsen claudication).

Many of these patients have generalised atheromatous vascular disease, and they have a high mortality from heart attack and stroke. All cardiovascular risk factors should be assessed and blood pressure should be controlled, and if serum cholesterol levels exceed 5.0 mmol/l, lipid-lowering agents should be prescribed. Smokers should be vehemently counselled on the importance of stopping.

Abdominal aortic aneurysm

There is a close association between hypertension and abdominal aneurysms, and some clinicians recommend the routine screening of all elderly symptomless hypertensive patients by abdominal ultrasound. If an aneurysm with a diameter greater than 6 cm is identified, elective surgical repair is worthwhile, as this procedure carries a much lower mortality than an emergency repair of a ruptured aneurysm. Careful control of blood pressure is mandatory to reduce the risk of rupture.

Claudication

All hypertensive patients and particularly those with calf pain should be examined for absent foot pulses and a femoral bruit. Many will also be found to have undiagnosed atheromatous renal artery stenosis (even if they are not hypertensive) so overenthusiastic drug therapy with large doses of ACE inhibitors can be hazardous. The calcium-channel blockers may help to reduce the severity of claudication. Diuretics do not make symptoms worse but in high doses may cause glucose intolerance and raise serum lipid levels. Beta-blockers may worsen the symptoms in patients with claudication, as well as causing cold extremities. However, they may have little influence on claudication distance, even though they do reduce cardiac output. There are case reports of gangrene induced by beta-blockers in patients with severe arterial disease.

Carotid artery disease

Patients who have had a TIA or a stroke may have extensive carotid atheroma. All should be assessed by carotid Doppler studies, and aspirin 75 mg daily should be prescribed. It should be remembered that the commonest cause of death in patients with TIA is due to a myocardial infarction. For this reason, all cardiovascular risk factors need to be assessed and managed as described earlier.

Raynaud's phenomenon

Although Raynaud's phenomenon is not associated with hypertension, where present it may be worsened by the use of beta-blockers. In such patients, these drugs are best avoided, but, if they are considered necessary, a beta-blocker that has intrinsic sympathomimetic activity (e.g. pindolol) is the most sensible choice as it will cause less reduction in cardiac output. ACE inhibitors, angiotensin-receptor antagonists or calcium-channel blockers are better options in such patients.

If a hypertensive patient has Raynaud's phenomenon, then a diagnosis of underlying scleroderma should be considered. There may be skin thickening, telangiectasia, subcutaneous calcinosis, a tight fissured appearance around the mouth and possibly symptoms of oesophageal involvement. In scleroderma, once the blood pressure becomes raised and there is renal involvement, the prognosis is poor as renal function deteriorates rapidly. There is some evidence that the ACE inhibitor captopril is effective in delaying further renal damage so this must be regarded as the first choice, possibly in conjunction with a calcium-channel blocker.

Cigarette smoking

Cigarette smoking really should be regarded as a disease and a dangerous one too. Many patients are severely addicted, it is now known, because the tobacco companies were adding extra nicotine. Clinicians should not therefore be judgemental of their patients who still smoke. Instead an active programme of education, with stopping smoking clinics, should be established. If the patient's cardiovascular status is stable, then nicotine chewing gum or patches are safe. The other cardiovascular risk factors should be treated aggressively in view of the heightened cardiovascular risk.

Renal disease

As stated in Chapter 7, patients with haematuria, proteinuria or renal impairment need detailed investigation. Many patients will be found to have intrinsic renal disease, including polycystic disease, IgA nephropathy, proliferative glomerulonephritis, polyarteritis and related conditions. However, a significant number of patients will be found to have no evidence of intrinsic renal disease and are considered to have hypertensive nephrosclerosis.

Intrinsic renal disease

Whilst raised blood pressure is not always found in patients with intrinsic renal disease, where present it substantially influences the prognosis both for the vascular complications of hypertension and for progression of renal impairment. Until recently, however, the evidence that antihypertensive therapy prevented progression of renal impairment was not impressive. However, there is now increasing evidence that good control of blood pressure slows down the deterioration of renal function in some cases. Two recent studies have compared an ACE inhibitor

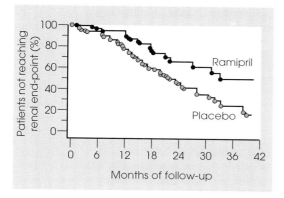

Figure 14.4

A comparison of the ACE inhibitor, ramipril, versus placebo in patients with non-diabetic nephropathy with 3 g/day or more proteinuria. A renal end point was defined as a doubling of serum creatinine or end-stage renal failure. Data from GISEN trial, 1997.

with other classes of antihypertensive drugs. Whilst there were no important differences in the antihypertensive effects, ACE inhibition caused significant reductions in either microproteinuria or macroproteinuria and there is now good evidence of preservation of renal function (Fig. 14.4). The evidence in favour of ACE inhibition in diabetics with renal impairment is also impressive.

Chronic renal failure

Most patients with chronic renal failure are hypertensive and the raised blood pressure sets up a vicious cycle, causing further renal damage. The patient is rendered clinically unwell, with anaemia, metabolic bone disease, pulmonary oedema and the general systemic effects of uraemia. At this late stage, dietary protein restriction and control of blood pressure may delay, but not prevent, the otherwise inexorable trend towards end-stage renal failure. Detailed investigation is still worthwhile, however, in order to exclude any underlying vasculitis, and if renal artery stenosis is present, its correction, either by surgery or angioplasty, may help to control blood pressure and preserve some renal function.

In chronic renal failure, those drugs that are excreted by the kidney need to be prescribed in much reduced doses. The hydrophilic beta-blockers, like atenolol, are frequently given on alternate days, and the doses of all ACE inhibitors need to be reduced because they can be hazardous if the patient becomes dehydrated, as they block any compensatory rise in plasma angiotensin II levels. The dihydropyridine calcium-channel blockers are effective when used with care. When there is sodium and water retention, loop diuretics like frusemide or bumetanide are used and large doses may be necessary.

Chronic dialysis

Once the patient is on chronic dialysis, either haemodialysis or chronic ambulatory peritoneal dialysis, hypertension is almost universal. Furthermore, the incidence of heart attacks and strokes is much higher than would be expected on the basis of the height of the blood pressure or the presence of other risk factors. In most patients, blood pressure can be controlled relatively easily by removing salt and water during dialysis. Between dialyses, restriction of salt and water can help to control the pressure, but in many patients antihypertensive drugs may be necessary.

In a small minority of patients with end-stage renal failure, the remnant chronically damaged kidneys substantially aggravate the hypertension. In these patients, the renin–angiotensin system becomes over-sensitive to sodium depletion. At the time of dialysis, plasma angiotensin II concentrations rise to very high levels and there is an intense vasoconstrictor-mediated rise in blood pressure. This rise in pressure can, in part, be controlled by drugs that either suppress renin release (beta-blockers) or inhibit the generation of angiotensin II (ACE inhibitors) combined usually with a calcium-channel blocker. Occasionally bilateral nephrectomy may be necessary.

Erythropoetin

The advent of erythropoetin for the correction of the normochromic normocytic anaemia of chronic renal failure has provided further problems in the control of blood pressure. The mechanisms of the erythropoetin-induced rise in blood pressure are complex. The rise in haematocrit as the anaemia improves may lead to a reduction of effective renal plasma flow, but erythropoetin may also have some properties in common with renin or angiotensin, acting as a direct vasoconstrictor. Whatever the mechanisms, when erythropoetin is given, the blood pressure should be carefully monitored and controlled with drugs if necessary.

Renal transplantation

Hypertension develops in around 75% of patients who have undergone renal transplantation and the reasons for this are complex. There is evidence that hypertension tends to follow the transplanted kidney. Hypertension is commoner in the recipient if the donor had hypertension or had a strong family history of hypertension. This finding has important implications for our understanding of the aetiology of essential hypertension and reflects the results of cross-transplantation experiments in rats.

In the early postoperative period, raised blood pressure may be due to the immediate host/transplant rejection reaction, with the development of renal damage and an increase in renin and angiotensin release. This hypertension may partly come under control with immunosuppressive therapy. There may, however, also be a volume expansion component to the raised blood pressure due to fluid overload prior to transplantation, or if the transplant itself is rejected, it fails to excrete sodium and water. This problem is further compounded by sodium and water retention caused by the high doses of corticosteroids used to suppress rejection.

The advent of cyclosporin has been a major advance in the prevention of transplant rejection, but cyclosporin itself can raise blood pressure. Cyclosporin is also associated with hypertension following bone marrow and cardiac transplants. The mechanism is uncertain but cyclosporin may have some direct vasoconstrictor properties, possibly potentiating the effects of renin and angiotensin.

Following renal transplantation, raised blood pressure may be further aggravated by excess renin release from the host's own failed kidneys. On a longer term basis, transplant recipients have a greatly increased tendency to develop generalised arteriosclerosis. Atheromatous renal artery stenosis is common in transplanted kidneys and this can contribute to the development of hypertension. Occasionally the anastomosis of transplanted renal artery becomes stenosed, causing severe elevation of blood pressure.

The accurate control of blood pressure is important following renal transplantation. All the main classes of antihypertensive drugs may be used, but renal failure may develop and doses of drugs may need to be adjusted. Acute deterioration of renal function may cause a sharp rise in serum potassium, particularly if patients are taking an ACE inhibitor.

DIABETES MELLITUS

The relationship between hypertension and the two forms of diabetes (type 1, insulin-dependent diabetes mellitus or IDDM and type II, non-insulin-dependent or NIDDM) is a close one, but this topic has, sadly, been neglected until recently.

Cardiovascular risk factors in diabetes

Hypertension is present in around 20% of patients with IDDM and 30–50% of patients with NIDDM. In patients of Afro-Caribbean origin the prevalence of raised blood pressure in NIDDM is even higher (Fig. 14.5).

It is also important to note that hyperlipidaemia occurs in NIDDM at about twice the frequency of that seen in the general population. Furthermore, cigarette smoking is also common. This means that all three cardiovascular risk factors tend to be very common in diabetics and frequently they assume greater prognostic importance than the severity of the diabetes itself. The slavish obsession with controlling blood sugar, particularly in NIDDM, whilst ignoring or not even measuring the other cardiovascular risk factors, has been a feature of many

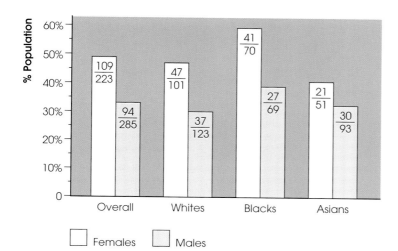

Figure 14.5
The prevalence of hypertension in white, black and Asian diabetics.

cattle-market style diabetic clinics in the past, and patients have suffered accordingly.

The aetiology of hypertension in diabetes

The pathophysiology of the association between hypertension and diabetes has been the focus of much research. It is probable that the mechanisms differ in IDDM versus NIDDM although there may be some overlap. In IDDM, where plasma insulin levels are low on a long-term basis, diabetic microangiopathy develops, and the raised blood pressure is mostly related to the development of diabetic nephrosclerosis with activation of the renin–angiotensin system and a largely vasoconstrictor-mediated hypertension. There may also be a contribution from sodium and water retention, although this is not apparent when estimating total exchangeable sodium or body water. By contrast, NIDDM is more closely related to volume expansion with increased total exchangeable sodium. Plasma renin and angiotensin levels are not usually high. This sodium retention is thought to be related to the degree of hyper-insulinaemia in NIDDM. In older patients with NIDDM, particularly if they are also cigarette smokers, there may be extensive large vessel atheroma, so atheromatous renal artery stenosis may contribute to the hypertension and renal impairment. Most patients with NIDDM are also obese and, even after correction for the tendency to overestimate blood pressure in obese arms, there remains a strong association between diabetes and hypertension.

Obesity itself is associated with hyperin-sulinaemia, which may itself be a factor in the development of raised blood pressure. The sulphonylurea drugs used in the treat-ment of NIDDM themselves cause weight gain and may aggravate the hypertension.

Insulin resistance

A unifying hypothesis to explain the concordance of hypertension, obesity, hypertriglyc-eridaemia and glucose intolerance has been put forward. It implies a prime role for insulin resistance and, therefore, hyperin-sulinaemia in the elevation of blood pressure. The mechanisms are uncertain but insulin itself is a vascular proliferative factor and, furthermore, under certain circumstances insulin causes fluid retention.

It was demonstrated many years ago that some non-obese, non-diabetic essential hypertensives have modest impairment of glucose tolerance, so they are mildly insulin resistant. The same phenomenon is seen in non-diabetic, non-hypertensive, obese individuals with a strong family history of hypertension. Could insulin resistance, therefore, be a final common pathway for the development of hypertension? However, if insulin resistance is an important mechanism in hypertension, then drugs that worsen insulin resistance would be expected to raise rather than lower blood pressure. This is clearly not so; the thiazides and, to a lesser extent, the beta-blockers have 'adverse' effects on insulin sensitivity but are very effective in lowering blood pressure, and thiazides are effective at preventing heart attacks and strokes. Manufacturers of the calcium-channel blockers and the ACE inhibitors are keen to point out that these drugs have no effects on glucose tolerance, but it remains uncertain whether this is an important consideration. The biguanide antidiabetic drugs, which improve insulin sensitivity, have no antihypertensive properties. The importance of insulin resistance appears to have been exaggerated.

Treating hypertension in IDDM

In view of the very poor outlook in patients with IDDM once they have developed hypertension, it is generally considered desirable to lower the threshold for starting antihypertensive drug therapy. If the systolic blood pressure exceeds 140 mmHg and/or the diastolic blood pressure exceeds 90 mmHg on four occasions, a few weeks apart, despite all the non-pharmacological manoeuvres outlined in Chapter 10, then antihypertensive drugs should be instituted. Thiazide diuretics are best avoided in view of their metabolic side-effects. Beta-blockers are generally safe but may cause problems in very 'brittle' diabetics with frequent episodes of insulin-induced hypoglycaemia. For this reason, the cardioselective beta-blockers, atenolol or metoprolol, are preferred.

Clinical experience with calcium-channel blockers and ACE inhibitors in diabetics is extensive. Both classes of drug have no adverse metabolic effects on glucose or lipid levels and when used carefully they are safe. The ACE inhibitors, in the long term, confer special advantages in IDDM as long as they are used prudently.

Treating hypertension in NIDDM

The topic of hypertension in patients with NIDDM was advanced in 1998 with the publication of the UK Prospective Diabetes Study (UK PDS) of blood pressure lowering. This demonstrated that tight control of blood pressure lead to significant reductions in diabetic endpoints, including death as well as strokes and the microvascular complications (retinopathy and nephropathy). There were also non-significant reductions in all-cause mortality, myocardial infarctions and peripheral vascular disease.

Tight control meant that the blood pressure had to be reduced to below 150/85 mmHg, and the average pressure at follow-up was 144/82 mmHg. The control group with less tight control of pressure had an average blood pressure of 154/87 mmHg at follow-up. The achieved blood pressure in the tight control group was remarkably close to the optimal blood pressure in the Hypertension Optimal Treatment (HOT) trial (see Chapter 9). One surprising finding of UK PDS was the lack of difference in outcome in patients randomised to atenolol compared with those given captopril.

It is important to note, also, that the benefits of tight control of blood pressure were greater than the benefits of attempts to achieve tight glycaemic control with antidiabetic drugs. This finding confirms the view that Type 2 diabetes should be considered as one of a cluster of cardiovascular risk factors and if hypertension is present, it should be treated aggressively.

All patients with NIDDM should be assessed carefully and blood pressure should be measured at every visit. Advice by a nutritionist is mandatory in all patients to reduce weight and restrict salt intake. Low-calorie fruit and vegetables should be substituted for convenience or processed foods. If the blood pressure remains over 140/90 mmHg, antihypertensive drugs should be prescribed, and the diastolic blood pressure reduced to below 80 mmHg (see Chapter 9, the results of the HOT trial).

Hypertension in patients with NIDDM may prove difficult to control. Beta-blockers and ACE inhibitors are suitable first-line agents but in most patients it is necessary to add in a long-acting calcium-channel blocker. Amlodipine rather than verapamil is best added to a beta-blocker but any calcium blocker can be used with an ACE inhibitor. Control of blood glucose of HbA_1C is also worthwhile and thiazides are not recommended routinely as they may interfere with glycaemic control.

Diabetes and serum cholesterol

The value of lipid lowering in diabetic patients has not yet been tested in formal clinical trials. However, in the Scandinavian Simvastatin Survival Study (SSSS), the patients surviving myocardial infarction who also had diabetes (mainly NIDDM) obtained particular benefits from cholesterol lowering. All diabetics with any degree of heart disease should be prescribed a statin if their serum cholesterol levels exceed 5.0 mmol/l. In diabetics without overt heart disease the threshold is uncertain, but we would prescribe a statin if the serum cholesterol exceeds 6.5 mmol/l.

Proteinuria and microproteinuria

The impact of antihypertensive drugs on renal function in diabetic patients is the focus of much research. Until recently, there was scant evidence that treating the hypertension or the diabetes had any impact on renal function. Once renal damage was present, it became progressively worse until the patient developed end-stage renal failure requiring dialysis or transplantation.

Once proteinuria on dipstick testing is present the outlook is poor, and there is now evidence that the presence of microproteinuria is also predictive but at an earlier stage. Microproteinuria is said to be present if the urine albumin concentration is between 30 and 300 mg/l, i.e. below the limit of urine dipstick sensitivity.

Well conducted, randomised trials in diabetic patients with proteinuria have shown that ACE inhibitors cause a significant reduction in urinary albumin excretion. Several trials have demonstrated a slowing of the rate of deterioration of renal function in patients on ACE inhibitors (Fig. 14.6). The beta-blockers and calcium-channel blockers, whilst equally effective at lowering blood pressure, showed less impressive or no effects on microproteinuria. Studies of the use of ACE inhibitors in diabetic patients

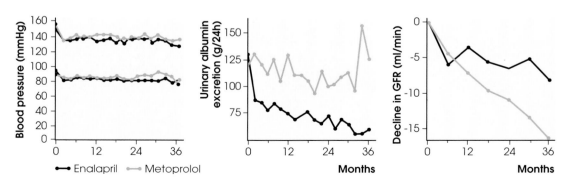

Figure 14.6
Comparison of enalapril and metoprolol in diabetic hypertensive patients with proteinuria.

with proteinuria but with normal blood pressure are now appearing and preliminary results look encouraging.

The reason why ACE inhibition appears to confer added benefits over other drugs for the same reduction in blood pressure may be related to the fall in angiotensin II levels, causing glomerular efferent arteriolar vasodilatation and a reduction in intraglomerular pressure.

There is now sufficient evidence to recommend the routine use of ACE inhibitors in all hypertensive patients with IDDM. Trials are now underway to investigate the value of the angiotensin-receptor antagonists in diabetic patients with subclinical or overt nephropathy. It is our practice to use these drugs in such patients if ACE inhibitors cause side-effects.

Diabetic retinopathy

There is now evidence that ACE inhibitors delay the progression of retinopathy in diabetic patients. This provides further powerful reasons to use these drugs as first line in patients with diabetes (IDDM or NIDDM) with blood pressure that consistently exceeds 140/90 mmHg.

HYPERTENSION AND HYPERLIPIDAEMIA

This topic is covered in other chapters but is sufficiently important to merit special mention here. In a hypertensive patient, if hyperlipidaemia is also present, with high

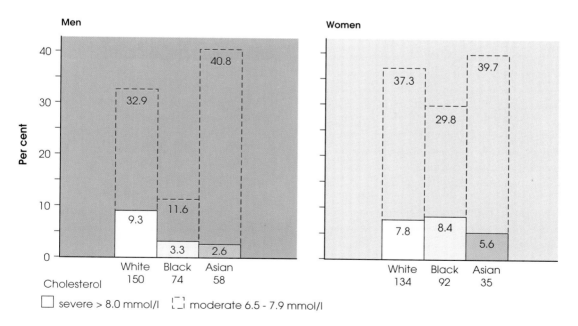

severe > 8.0 mmol/l   moderate 6.5 - 7.9 mmol/l

Figure 14.7
The prevalence of moderate and severe hypercholesterolaemia in a hypertension clinic.

blood cholesterol levels and low HDL cholesterol levels, the risk of coronary heart disease is greatly increased.

Serum cholesterol levels of 8 mmol/l or more are seen in 8–10% of hypertensive patients (Fig. 14.7). Cholesterol levels above 6.5 mmol/l are seen in a further 20%. All hypertensive patients should be considered to be at high risk and have routine serum cholesterol testing. Dietetic treatment of hypertensive patients with raised or even borderline serum cholesterol levels is mandatory.

The whole topic of cholesterol lowering has been transformed since 1995 with the publication of the SSSS Trial and the West of Scotland Coronary Prevention Group Study (WOSCOPS). Until these randomised controlled trials were published there was considerable uncertainty of the value of cholesterol-lowering drugs, and even some anxieties that they might be hazardous. However, these two studies convincingly showed that cholesterol lowering with an HMG CoA reductase inhibitor (a statin) caused a highly significant reduction of both first and recurrent myocardial infarction and death. Furthermore, in the SSSS trial there was a significant reduction in stroke rates. In the WOSCOPS study, the benefits of a statin in patients with serum cholesterol levels of about 7.0 mmol/l or higher were greater than the benefits of treating the milder grades of hypertension.

The implications of the two trials described above have still not sufficiently filtered down into clinical practice. In our view, however, urgent action is now needed to lower cholesterol levels in almost all hypertensive patients initially by dietary means. Where dietary manoeuvres do not control cholesterol, then we recommend the use of one of the statin group of lipid-lowering agents. The question is what is the threshold for introducing these drugs.

We strongly recommend the use of a statin in practically all patients with any degree of coronary heart disease and cholesterol levels exceeding 5.0 mmol/l.

In hypertensive patients who do not have any coronary disease the threshold is uncertain, but it is our practice to prescribe a statin in all patients with serum cholesterol levels of 6.5 mmol/l or more. The question of what to do with cholesterol levels between 5.0 and 6.5 mmol/l is the focus of the Anglo–Scandinavian Cardiac Outcome Trial (ASCOT), which was established in 1998. Until the results of this study are published, we recommend lipid-lowering agents in all hypertensive patients found to be at high cardiovascular risk by virtue of a bad family history of heart disease, the presence of LVH on the ECG or any evidence of non-cardiac atheromatous disease including stroke or peripheral vascular disease.

HYPERTENSION AND UNRELATED CONCOMITANT DISEASE

A great many hypertensive patients have other medical problems that substantially influence the choice of antihypertensive drugs. This problem, like hypertension itself, becomes commoner with advancing age. Often the concomitant disease is more important than the height of the blood pressure, so the clinician must balance the risks and benefits of treatment, taking into account the absolute risk of heart attack or stroke for his or her individual patient.

Asthma

In patients with any form of obstructive airways disease, beta-blockers are absolutely

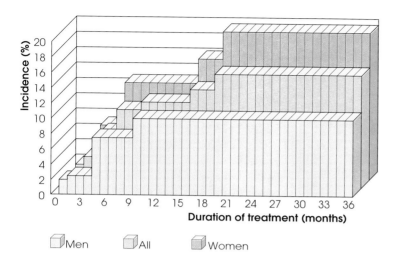

Figure 14.8
The incidence of cough in hypertensive patients receiving enalapril.

☐ Men   ☐ All   ☐ Women

contraindicated. This is true for the third-generation beta-blockers like celiprolol or bisoprolol although they do cause less bronchoconstriction than the earlier agents. Airways resistance is related to β2–adrenergic function and beta-blockade makes things worse; these drugs may interfere with the action of the β2–agonist inhalers like salbutamol.

All other antihypertensive drugs can be used safely and have no impact on airways resistance.

Patients on chronic low-dose corticosteroid therapy for asthma probably do not sustain a significant rise in blood pressure, although they do need careful monitoring. Short courses of high doses of prednisolone for acute asthma can cause elevation of blood pressure, but the hazards of this are greatly outweighed by the benefits of steroids in saving the lives of severe asthmatics.

Steroid therapy and beta agonists both tend to lower serum potassium levels, which may be predictive of a poorer outcome in acute asthma. In patients who also have hypertension, the thiazide diuretics, which also lower serum potassium levels, should be used with caution. If persistent hypokalaemia is encountered, however, a diagnosis of primary aldosteronism should be considered.

Cough

There are no significant adverse effects of ACE inhibitors on airways resistance. However, ACE inhibitors cause an irritating dry cough in about 10% of patients (Fig. 14.8). Middle-aged female non-smokers are particularly prone to develop this problem. Cough may also be an early symptom of asthma, so such patients require careful assessment. If a cough develops with one ACE inhibitor, it will almost certainly occur with all others, so this class of drug has to be abandoned. The cough may take up to 6 weeks to abate following cessation of ACE inhibition. It is now clear that the angiotensin-receptor antagonists do not have this side-effect. If the cough does not go away, then ACE inhibitors were not the cause; more detailed respiratory tests are necessary and ACE inhibitors may be restarted with caution.

Clinicians must be aware that the ACE inhibitors can cause acute angioedema with swelling of the lips and tongue and laryngeal stridor. This is most commonly seen in black patients.

Gastrointestinal symptoms

Many drugs may cause postprandial epigastric discomfort, but this side-effect is sporadic and idiosyncratic. Only spironolactone persistently causes indigestion.

Constipation commonly develops in patients taking verapamil in particular, but also with the other calcium-channel blockers. If alteration of bowel habit persists, despite stopping verapamil, detailed gastrointestinal investigation is mandatory.

Dentists should be aware that all the dihydropyridine calcium-channel blockers can cause gum hypertrophy, particularly if there is poor dental hygiene.

Liver disease

Patients with liver disease generally do not have hypertension, but the association of alcoholism, raised blood pressure and stroke is important. Abnormal liver function tests with raised gamma glutamyl transferase levels strongly suggest this diagnosis. In cirrhosis of the liver, ACE inhibitors may be hazardous. Those ACE inhibitors that are hepatically metabolised (e.g. enalapril, metabolised to enalaprilat) may be less effective if there is impairment of hepatic function.

Urogenital disease

Sexual function

Impotence is common in anxious hypertensive patients. The thiazide diuretics are an important cause of impotence and should be avoided in sexually active men. Beta-blockers may also cause impotence, but there appear to be no consistent effects on sexual function with ACE inhibitors or the calcium-channel blockers. The alpha-blockers are probably the best choice for men with problems with sexual function as they may improve things. Now that drugs are available that do not affect sexual function, the clinician should specifically enquire about this topic and choose antihypertensive therapy accordingly. There is no evidence that any antihypertensive drug adversely affects fertility.

Prostatism

Patients with symptoms of prostatic obstruction need careful urological assessment. Alpha-blockers may relieve symptoms a little, pending prostatectomy. Thus, these are logical drugs to use in men with hypertension and mild symptoms of prostatic enlargement. The dihydropyridine calcium antagonists such as nifedipine often cause nocturia, which needs to be distinguished from symptoms of prostatic enlargement.

Incontinence

Patients receiving the loop diuretic frusemide may develop urgency of micturition, and female patients may develop urge or stress incontinence. Loop diuretics should be avoided, particularly in women with a tendency to problems with control of bladder function. Many female patients have stress incontinence but are embarrassed to mention this to their cardiovascular specialist.

The alpha-blocking agents prazocin, doxazocin and terazocin may cause or aggravate stress incontinence in women. This symptom may not be volunteered by the patient so specific enquiry is recommended so that, if necessary, alternative antihypertensive drugs can be used.

The menopause

Blood pressure tends to rise in women after the menopause, so careful monitoring of blood pressure is advised. Hormone replacement therapy (HRT) is not contraindicated in hypertensive women but is best not given until the blood pressure is controlled; if it is given, regular 3-monthly checks are necessary. No consistent tendency of HRT to cause raised blood pressure has been documented and it may even improve control of hypertension in some women.

CONNECTIVE TISSUE DISEASES

Systemic lupus erythematosus, polyarteritis nodosa, mixed connective disease and progressive systemic sclerosis (scleroderma) are all associated with renal damage and hypertension. Furthermore, corticosteroid therapy for these conditions can further elevate blood pressure. Antihypertensive drugs are often necessary and calcium-channel blockers or ACE inhibitors are the most suitable agents. There is some evidence that ACE inhibitors have specific protective effects on the kidney in scleroderma.

Many drugs used by rheumatologists to relieve joint pains (e.g. ibuprofen or naproxen) or influence the progression of rheumatoid arthritis (e.g. indomethacin, gold or corticosteroids) can elevate blood pressure or interfere with antihypertensive drugs. A balance has to be struck between the harmful effects of these drugs on blood pressure and the benefits of pain relief and rheumatoid disease limitation.

Indomethacin is only indicated in the acute phases of gout and, in the long term, for the inflammatory arthritides; it should not be used routinely for degenerative joint disease.

Gout

Hyperuricaemia and gout may be a mendelian dominant condition or may be associated with hypertension, alcohol abuse, renal failure or the thiazide diuretics. Mildly elevated uric acid levels are common in hypertension and should not be treated with allopurinol.

ANAESTHESIA

Patients who undergo surgery when they have diastolic blood pressures persistently in excess of 120 mmHg have a higher incidence of intra-operative or postoperative cardiac arrhythmias or myocardial infarction. This is often associated with concomitant coronary artery or generalised vascular disease. For this reason, elective surgery should not be carried out in these patients until they are fully assessed and the blood pressure controlled. The moments of greatest cardiovascular risk are during laryngoscopy and intubation, during hypotensive anaesthesia to aid haemostasis, and whilst the surgeon is manipulating the abdominal viscera. Spinal anaesthesia can cause profound hypotension.

Sudden withdrawal of beta-blocking drugs in patients with established coronary artery disease may cause exacerbation of angina, and these drugs should not be stopped in the peri-operative period. The anaesthetist must be aware when a patient is taking antihypertensive drugs: they may impair the physiological responses to blood loss. In particular, beta-blockers will block the increase in heart rate that occurs with fluid loss, ACE inhibitors will block the compensatory response of the renin system, and, in some cases, with severe fluid loss hypotension may occur.

In the postoperative phase, while patients are resting in bed receiving pain-relieving drugs, blood pressure usually remains low. Antihypertensive drugs should be restarted as soon as the blood pressure rises again and the patient is able to swallow them. Before this time, while the patient is receiving intravenous fluids only, intramuscular antihypertensive drugs are very occasionally needed to control very high blood pressure.

Mild symptomless hypertension in an otherwise fit middle-aged person does not carry any excess cardiovascular risk during the pre-, intra- or postoperative period. All too often, inexperienced anaesthetists needlessly cancel elective surgery on account of trivial hypertension or often a transient elevation of blood pressure on hospital admission in an anxious patient. If the patient is allowed to relax, careful measurement of the blood pressure may reveal much lower pressures and the surgical procedure can go ahead, particularly if the ECG shows no evidence of LVH or ischaemia.

GLAUCOMA

Rapid falls in blood pressure may aggravate glaucoma. Thus, antihypertensive therapy should be given with care in patients with this condition. Beta-blockers are given topically to treat glaucoma, and a sufficient amount of the drug may be absorbed to induce systemic beta-blockade with some reduction of blood pressure.

PSYCHIATRIC DISEASE

Alcoholism

Alcoholics and heavy drinkers are more likely to be hypertensive than the general population and they should have their blood pressure monitored regularly, as they are particularly prone to develop strokes. See Chapters 3 and 10.

Anxiety states

Anxious patients may develop transiently raised blood pressure, particularly with high systolic pressures. There is, however, no evidence that chronic anxiety is a cause of hypertension. In anxious patients treatment of the underlying psychiatric disease should be instituted, but because of the mild anxiolytic effects of beta-blockers these may be employed if the patient is truly hypertensive.

The lipophilic beta-blockers like propranolol are effective in relieving symptoms of anxiety, as they freely enter the brain. Atenolol is only very slightly lipophilic but it does have some useful effects in very tense and anxious patients.

Depressive disease

Once patients have been told they are hypertensive, they may develop anxiety or depression about their condition. These problems may be compounded by the use of the centrally acting drugs (methyldopa, clonidine and reserpine), which can cause depression. These drugs should never be used in depressed patients and are best avoided in all other patients. Beta-blockers do not cause depression but they may induce lethargy. This problem is particularly seen with propranolol, oxprenolol, metoprolol and timolol, but possibly less with atenolol or nadolol. ACE inhibitors and angiotensin-receptor antagonists, with their complete absence of central side-effects, makes them potentially useful in depressed patients; the calcium-channel blockers are also useful.

In patients with bipolar depression or manic depressive psychosis, psychiatrists commonly use lithium therapy. If the patient is also hypertensive, thiazide diuretics are specifically contraindicated as they may cause a dangerous rise in plasma lithium levels. There are reports of a rise in serum lithium levels in some patients receiving ACE inhibitors.

CONCLUSIONS

It will be seen from this chapter that the management of hypertension is relevant to practically all branches of the medical and nursing professions. Specialists who do not have a prime interest in hypertension all too frequently neglect their patients' blood pressure or manage it inefficiently or incorrectly. Improved awareness of the importance of hypertension as a major cause of death or disability and of the sensible choice of antihypertensive drugs can greatly benefit hypertensive patients who have concomitant medical conditions.

FURTHER READING

Barnett AH. Diabetes and hypertension. *Br Med Bull* 1994; **50**: 397–407.

Brown MA, Whitworth J. Hypertension in human renal disease. *J Hypertens* 1992; **10**: 701–12.

Chaturvedi N, Sjolie A-K, Stephenson JM. Effect of lisinopril on progression of retinopathy in normotensive people with type 1 diabetes. *Lancet* 1998; **351**: 28–31.

The GISEN Group (Gruppo Italiano di Studi Epidemiologici in Nephrologia). Randomised placebo controlled trial of effect of ramipril on decline in glomerular filtration rate and risk of terminal renal failure in proteinuric, non-diabetic nephropathy. *Lancet* 1997; **349**: 1857–63.

Lewis EJ, Hunsicker LG, Bain RP, *et al.* The effect of angiotensin-converting-enzyme inhibition on diabetic nephropathy. *N Engl J Med* 1993; **329**: 1456–62.

Lip GYH, Beevers M, Churchill D, *et al.* Hormone replacement therapy and blood pressure in hypertensive women. *J Hum Hypertens* 1994; **8**: 491–4.

O'Connell JE, Gray C. Treating hypertension after stroke. *Br Med J* 1994; **308**: 152–4.

Prys-Roberts C. Anaesthesia and hypertension. *Br J Anaesth* 1984; **56**: 711–24.

Reaven GM. Role of insulin resistance in human disease: Banting Lecture. *Diabetes* 1988; **37**: 1595–1607.

Scandinavian Simvastatin Survival Study Group. Randomized trial of cholesterol lowering in 4444 patients with coronary heart disease. *Lancet* 1994; **344**: 1383–9.

Shepherd J, Cobbe SM, Ford I, *et al.* Prevention of coronary heart disease with pravastatin in men with hypercholesterolemia. *N Engl J Med* 1995; **333**: 1301–7.

Turner RC, Millns H, Neil HAW, *et al.* Risk factors for coronary artery disease in non-insulin dependent diabetes mellitus: United Kingdom prospective diabetes study. (UKPDS:23) *Br Med J* 1998; **316**: 323–8.

UK Prospective Diabetes Study Group. Tight blood pressure control and risk of macrovascular and microvascular complications in type 2 diabetes: UKPDS 38. *Br Med J* 1998; **317**: 703–13.

Weston CFM, Penny WJ, Julian DG, on behalf of the British Heart Foundation Working Group. Guidelines for the early management of patients with myocardial infarction. *Br Med J* 1994; **308**: 767–71.

Winocour PH. Microalbuminuria: worth screening for in early morning urine samples in diabetic, hypertensive, and elderly patients. *Br Med J* 1992; **304**: 1196–7.

15 HYPERTENSION IN THE ELDERLY

BACKGROUND

In all the developed societies that consume large amounts of salt, blood pressure rises with advancing age. As a result, in an aging society, the number of people with high blood pressure increases unless they die prematurely from cardiovascular disease. If high blood pressure is defined as systolic blood pressure greater than 160 mmHg or diastolic pressure greater than 90 mmHg, then over half the population over the age of 65 will be considered to have hypertension.

For many years it was felt that older patients 'needed' their higher pressures to perfuse narrowed and stiffened arteries. This concept is totally incorrect. The risk of cardiovascular disease up to the age of 80 years from high blood pressure is identical to that in younger patients. Indeed, the actual or absolute risk of dying from a vascular event related to high blood pressure is greater in the elderly because the chance of developing a stroke or a heart attack rises as one gets older. In spite of this knowledge, it was argued that treatment of high blood pressure in the elderly was not justified because there was no evidence that treatment was beneficial. However, several recent trials have now unequivocally demonstrated the immense benefit of lowering blood pressure in the elderly. Antihypertension treatment provides greater benefit in the short term in the prevention of strokes, heart attacks and heart failure than in younger patients. Older patients with hypertension, at least up to the age of 80 years, must receive treatment. However, care needs to be taken in the choice of the drugs, using lower doses and avoiding those that cause postural drops in blood pressure.

THE RISE IN BLOOD PRESSURE WITH AGE

As pointed out earlier, blood pressure rises with age in developed societies. The rise in the systolic pressure tends to be greater than the rise in diastolic pressure and, in many patients, diastolic pressure may fall after the age of 65 years, giving rise to a widened pulse pressure. However, epidemiological evidence clearly shows that the systolic pressure is a very potent predictor of risk for coronary heart disease, heart failure and stroke over the age of 45 years irrespective of the diastolic pressure. It comes as a surprise to many clinicians that the systolic blood pressure is a more accurate predictor of risk than the diastolic pressure. Patients with isolated systolic hypertension with diastolic pressures below 90 mmHg have a poor prognosis but obtain great benefit from antihypertensive therapy.

ASSESSMENT OF THE PATIENT

In the majority of elderly patients, blood pressure measurement is straightforward. However, in a few, there may be a more pronounced systolic silent gap between the second and third Korotkoff phases, so systolic pressure may be underestimated if the cuff is not inflated to a level that occludes the radial pulse.

Elderly patients are more likely to have concomitant disease, either related to the hypertension, (e.g. coronary heart disease, heart failure, previous ischaemic or cerebrovascular disease), or other conditions unrelated to the blood pressure, including chronic chest disease, cancer and arthritis. Furthermore, NIDDM is commoner in the elderly. Clearly, in assessing these patients one needs to be careful not to miss these other important concomitant diseases that may need drug treatment. They may influence the choice of antihypertensive agents due to specific indications or contraindications.

Important changes occur in the elderly that influence the choice of drug treatment. There is a gradual reduction in glomerular filtration rate as age increases, so that renal function declines. On average, at the age of 70 years, renal function is about half that of a younger person. Therefore, drugs that are excreted or metabolized by the kidney tend to accumulate, and dosage adjustments must be made. Elderly patients also tend to have a less reactive renin system, and this results in their blood pressure being more responsive to changes in volume, particularly when diuretics or salt restriction are used. Furthermore, the lower levels of plasma renin and angiotensin in older patients will mean that drugs that work by blocking the renin system (e.g ACE inhibitors) tend to be less effective.

Elderly patients often have some impairment of the postural reflexes that maintain blood pressure on standing. This may lead, in some patients, to postural drops in blood pressure, even without antihypertensive drugs, which may be worsened when medication is started.

SECONDARY CAUSES OF HYPERTENSION IN THE ELDERLY

Secondary causes of hypertension in the elderly are just as common as in younger patients, contrary to what many experts have said in the past. Nevertheless, as in younger patients, the majority do not have an underlying cause and these patients are classified as having essential hypertension. However, routine investigations need to be done to exclude adrenal adenomas (low plasma potassium), and in those where there is severe hypertension or any unusual story that suggests a diagnosis of phaeochromocytomas (24-hour urinary catecholamine excretion). By far the most common cause of secondary hypertension in the elderly is renal artery stenosis related to generalized peripheral vascular disease. These patients usually are or have been heavy cigarette smokers. They usually have some degree of renal impairment and evidence of peripheral vascular disease with intermittent claudication, absent pulses in the legs, or evidence of ischaemic heart disease or cerebrovascular disease.

INVESTIGATIONS IN THE ELDERLY HYPERTENSIVE

The same routine investigations for younger patients described in Chapter 7 should also be done in the elderly. Clearly it is important to check kidney function with serum urea, creatinine and electrolyte levels. Heart failure tends to be common in these patients due to a combination of ischaemic heart disease and high blood pressure, so an ECG is mandatory and echocardiography may be necessary. Patients in whom renal artery stenosis is suspected should be referred to a specialised centre, as investigation, usually with a renal angiogram, carries some risks and is only justified where there is worsening renal function, uncontrollable hypertension or heart failure that may be secondary to the renal artery stenosis.

EVIDENCE FOR THE BENEFIT OF TREATMENT IN THE ELDERLY

Until recently there was some doubt about how beneficial it was to treat elderly hypertensive patients, as previous studies such as Hamilton's classic trial in 1964 in severe hypertensive patients and the Veteran's Administration trials with more moderate hypertension included only a few patients over the age of 60 years, and it was unclear whether this group did specifically benefit from treatment. Other evidence from the HDFP study and the Australian National High Blood Pressure trial did suggest that the elderly might benefit from treatment. However, recently several well conducted randomised controlled studies in the elderly have clearly demonstrated the immense benefits of drug treatment. The treatment trials in the elderly are discussed in more detail in Chapter 9.

The European Working Party on Hypertension in the Elderly (EWPHE) 1985 and the Coope and Warrender Trial 1985

The EWPHE trial was a large hospital-based study in patients over the age of 60 years who were randomised either to receive a thiazide diuretic combined with triamterene or a placebo. The study showed that blood pressure could be lowered without significant adverse effects, although there were some metabolic problems with the thiazide diuretics. Patients were included if they had systolic pressures of 160–239 mmHg and diastolic pressures of 90–119 mmHg. The study clearly demonstrated a reduction in cardiovascular and cerebrovascular mortality. At around the same time, Coope and Warrender conducted a similar trial in general practice in the UK, where patients were randomised either to a beta-blocker or to observation only. This showed similar results, with a reduction in strokes but no effect on coronary disease. There was no

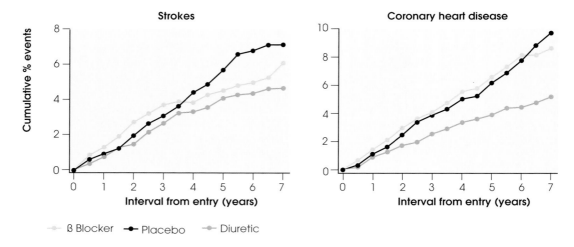

Figure 15.1
Results of treatment in the MRC trial of hypertension in the elderly.

reduction in total mortality rates from all causes even when the results of the two trials were combined.

Medical Research Council study in the elderly 1992

This was a randomised study in patients aged 65–74 years. Entry criteria included diastolic pressures of less than 115 mmHg, and systolic pressures of 160–204 mmHg. The study was a comparison of the beta-blocker atenolol or a diuretic against placebo and included over 4,000 patients. The study clearly demonstrated the benefit of treatment in the elderly. Diuretics, in particular, reduced cerebrovascular strokes, but did not reduce coronary heart disease (Fig. 15.1). The exact reasons for this are not clear and have been disputed. However, what is clear is that beta-blockers were not as effective in lowering blood pressure as

the diuretics, and this may explain why they prevented fewer heart attacks.

Swedish Trial of Old Patients with Hypertension (STOP-H) 1991

This trial from Sweden again clearly demonstrated the benefits of treatment in elderly hypertensive patients with either a beta-blocker or a diuretic. A sub-group analysis of the two different treatments has not been published so it is impossible to say whether one form of therapy is better than any other in this particular study.

Systolic Hypertension in the Elderly Program (SHEP) 1991

This study was specifically set up to look at elderly patients who had raised systolic

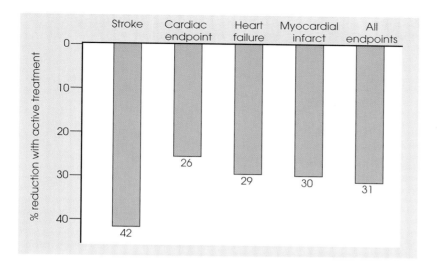

Figure 15.2
Detailed results of the Syst-Eur Trial (1997).

	AUST	EWPHE	COOPE	SHEP	STOP	MRC	SYST-EUR
Stroke	-34	-36*	-42*	-32*	-47*	-25*	-42*
Cardiac	-19	-20	-15	-27*	-13	-19	-26
Deaths	-23	-9	-3	-13	-43*	-3	-14

*p <0.05

Figure 15.3
Percentage change in events' in randomised controlled trials in the elderly.

pressure with normal diastolic pressure. In order to recruit these patients a very large number of people had to be screened, and the patients who were eventually studied were a very highly selected group of people who had isolated systolic hypertension but who were otherwise well. The trial was a randomised controlled study using the thiazide-like diuretic, chlorthalidone, with a beta-blocker added in if the blood pressure was not controlled. This regime was compared with placebo tablets. The study clearly demonstrated a significant reduction in strokes and coronary heart disease. In the placebo group the average systolic blood pressure after the run-in phase of the study showed an average systolic pressure of 155 mmHg, whilst in the actively treated group average systolic pressures were reduced to 144 mmHg. The mean on-treatment diastolic pressures in the placebo and active groups were 71 mmHg and 68 mmHg respectively.

Before accepting these entry levels of blood pressure and assuming that the whole of this elderly population should be treated, it should be remembered that these were highly selected patients. Nevertheless, the trial did show that even quite mild degrees of isolated systolic hypertension in the elderly, which carry an increased risk of cerebrovascular and cardiovascular disease, are worth reducing.

European Trial of Systolic Hypertension in the Elderly (SYST-EUR) 1997

The details of the SYST-EUR trial are described in more detail in Chapter 9. This important study confirmed, without any shadow of doubt, that isolated systolic hypertension in the elderly is worth treating (Fig. 15.2). It also showed that the newer antihypertensive drugs, the calcium-channel blockers and the ACE inhibitors, are quite as effective as the thiazide diuretics at preventing heart attacks and strokes. Furthermore, there was no 'downside' with increased morbidity from symptoms, side-effects or non-cardiovascular disease.

An overview of all of the blood pressure-lowering trials in the elderly is shown in Figure 15.3. The reduction in stroke was significant in all the trials. When all the data are pooled, the reduction in strokes, coronary disease and death from all causes reaches statistical significance.

INDICATIONS FOR ANTIHYPERTENSIVE TREATMENT IN ELDERLY PATIENTS

Taking into account all the trials described above, there is no doubt that it is very beneficial to treat hypertension in the elderly. There are still some open questions, particularly over the age of 80 years and in mild degrees of isolated systolic hypertension. Balanced against the benefits of treatment there must be consideration of the problems of the organisation and administration of antihypertensive treatment in the elderly, and the possible side-effects of the drugs. However, the incidence of serious side-effects in the SHEP and SYST-EUR studies was remarkably low.

Accelerated hypertension or very severe hypertension

This syndrome is not as uncommon as previously thought and should always be treated, irrespective of age. As in the younger population, very good results can be obtained with accurate blood pressure control. However, in this group it is particularly important to avoid over-rapid reduction of blood pressure as this may cause cerebral or myocardial infarction. The high risk of there being underlying atheromatous renal artery stenosis means that ACE inhibitors should be avoided until this diagnosis is excluded. The optimum first-line drug is nifedipine in the 20 mg tablet formulation twice daily.

Patients with hypertension and congestive heart failure

These patients should always be treated, as the lowering of blood pressure may bring about relief of their heart failure. ACE inhibitors should be introduced with great caution, but in the longer term these drugs are very effective at preventing death in patients with heart failure at all ages.

Patients up to the age of 80 years

If the diastolic pressure, in spite of non-pharmacological advice, remains consistently over 90 mmHg, then antihypertensive drugs should be given, provided there are no obvious contraindications. Systolic pressure should also be reduced if it is consistently greater than 160 mmHg. It is worth pointing out to these patients that the control of blood pressure is highly effective at preventing strokes, which are the complications of hypertension particularly dreaded by elderly patients. The threshold for starting drug treatment is reduced to 140/90 mmHg if there is concurrent diabetes mellitus, according to some experts, although there is no randomised trial evidence to support this view.

Patients over the age of 80 years

In those studies that included some patients over the age of 80 years there were benefits in both stroke and heart attack prevention, although the numbers were quite small. There is no reason why these older patients should not benefit from reduction in blood pressure, but in view of the limited evidence it is probably better to only treat those whose systolic pressure is greater than 180 mmHg or whose diastolic pressure is greater than 95 mmHg. Patients already on treatment should not have treatment stopped just because they have reached the age of 80. The benefits of treating hypertension in the very old are currently being investigated in a randomised placebo-controlled trial in Europe (HYVET, see Chapter 9). It should be noted, however, that the small sub-set of patients in the SHEP trial who were aged over 80 years did derive as much benefit in terms of stroke prevention as the younger participants.

DOES TREATMENT OF THE ELDERLY DIFFER FROM THAT OF YOUNGER PATIENTS?

Non-pharmacological treatment

All patients should be advised about non-pharmacological treatment in the same way as in younger patients (see Chapter 10).

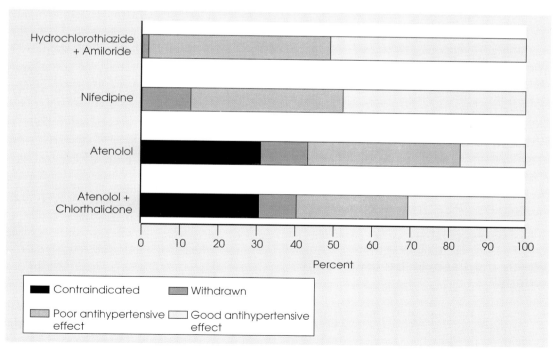

Figure 15.4

Drugs in the treatment of isolated systolic hypertension. (From Avanzini, et al. Eur Heart J 1994; **14**: 206–12).

Reduction of salt intake is particularly effective in older patients in view of their less reactive renin–angiotensin system. Many older patients tend to take large amounts of the salt in their food and may initially find it difficult to reduce this due to a decrease in the sensitivity of salt receptors in the mouth with increasing age. Our experience, however, is that if careful explanation is given and if patients are told that it will take them a few weeks to adjust, they will find that they get used to less salty foods and, after a while, may prefer them. The problem is that only between 10 and 20% of the total amount of salt consumed is added in cooking or at table. The remainder is added to food by the manufacturers so that they can add more water and thus increase bulk. This is a particular problem in convenience foods, including sausages and canned meats, which many elderly people tend to rely on.

Many elderly patients consume inadequate amounts of potassium-rich food and it is important therefore to try and encourage a greater consumption of fresh fruit and vegetables. This particularly applies if thiazide diuretics are being given. There is some epidemiological evidence that elderly people who consume a diet low in potassium have an increased risk of stroke. Excess weight and excess alcohol should clearly be dealt with in the same way as in younger patients.

Which drug should be used in the elderly?

In general terms, the same drugs are used as in younger patients. However, lower doses should be used initially owing to a decreased clearance or metabolism of the drugs by the liver and kidneys with increasing age. There

are some age-related differences in drug response, largely related to the fact that elderly patients tend to have lower plasma renin and angiotensin levels, which are less responsive to changes in intravascular volume (Fig. 15.4).

Thiazide diuretics

Most of the controlled randomised trials in the elderly used the thiazide diuretics as first-line agents and there is no doubt that they do reduce both strokes and, perhaps surprisingly, coronary heart disease. Low-dose thiazide diuretics are particularly effective in the elderly and have the advantage that they have fewer metabolic side-effects. However, these should be looked for. Hypokalaemia is particularly important as many old people tend to consume inadequate amounts of potassium in their diet. Whether it is justified to add a potassium-sparing diuretic such as amiloride or triamterene to the diuretic is a matter of debate. In our view it is better not to do this unless the plasma potassium falls. Salt restriction will also prevent large falls in plasma potassium. Thiazide diuretics may occasionally cause postural drops in blood pressure. Thiazides may worsen glucose intolerance and this may contraindicate or limit their use in elderly patients who have both hypertension and NIDDM.

Beta-blockers

Beta-blockers on their own are less effective at lowering blood pressure in the elderly. However, the trials in the elderly do seem to indicate that, when combined with a thiazide diuretic beta-blockers have an additive effect and are useful. Low doses of these drugs should be given, as with the thiazide diuretics (Fig. 15.4). They are more likely to cause problems with peripheral blood flow and in patients with peripheral vascular disease they are best avoided. Many elderly patients complain of cold hands and feet on beta-blockers, and the insidious side-effects of lethargy, sleep disturbance and reduced exercise tolerance are common in the elderly as in younger patients. The use of beta-blockers is declining in all age groups as a result of these insidious and mildly debilitating side-effects.

ACE inhibitors

The ACE inhibitors when used alone tend to be less effective in older patients. Nevertheless, when combined with a thiazide diuretic or a calcium-channel blocker, they become effective, especially if also combined with a low-salt diet. These drugs are particularly useful in congestive heart failure in the elderly. However, patients who smoke and have evidence of peripheral vascular disease may also have renal artery stenosis where ACE inhibitors can cause a deterioration in renal function. It is essential in these patients that renal function is checked before and after 2 or 3 weeks if an ACE inhibitor is used.

As stated earlier, both hypertension and non-insulin dependent diabetes mellitus are common in the elderly, particularly where there is associated obesity. When these two conditions co-exist, the risk of heart attack, stroke and renal damage is greatly increased.

There is now an increasing body of evidence that ACE inhibitors are more effective than other antihypertensive drugs at delaying further deterioration in renal function in patients with both non-diabetic and diabetic nephropathy. This means that ACE inhibitors are probably specifically indicated in elderly patients with hypertension and diabetes mellitus. However, these drugs should be introduced gradually, with regular monitoring of blood pressure and renal function.

Angiotensin-receptor antagonists

The first angiotensin-receptor antagonist, losartan, was introduced in 1995, and many more drugs in this group will become available over the next few years. There is as yet very little information on their use in the elderly. In one clinical trial, losartan was compared with the long-acting formulation of the calcium-channel blocker, felodipine; it appeared to be minimally less effective but had fewer side-effects.

In view of the similarity of action of these drugs to the ACE inhibitors, the indications and possible hazards (e.g. in patients with concomitant renal artery stenosis) still apply. Angiotensin-receptor antagonists are remarkably free of side-effects and do not cause cough or angioedema. They can therefore be used in elderly patients where ACE inhibitors have caused these side-effects.

Only one long-term outcome trial of losartan is available and that was in elderly patients with mild heart failure (the ELITE trial). In this study losartan appeared to be somewhat more effective than captopril with a modestly lower mortality rate from sudden death and myocardial infarction. At the present state of knowledge, these agents can be used in the elderly with heart failure where ACE inhibitors have caused side-effects.

Calcium-channel blockers

These drugs, like the diuretics, appear on their own to be effective in the elderly and are used as initial treatment in exactly the same way as in younger patients, but again lower doses should be used at first. Anxieties about long-term side-effects of calcium-channel blockers have largely been allayed by the results of the SYST-EUR trial.

FIRST- AND SECOND-LINE AGENTS

It is our policy to use thiazide diuretics in low dose as first-line drugs in elderly patients. In the large proportion of patients where thiazides are contraindicated, we use the long-acting calcium-channel blockers (amlodipine, slow-release verapamil or nifedipine LA) instead. We only use beta-blockers as first-line agents where there is concomitant angina pectoris and we prefer to use them in low doses. Beta-blockers are not the best first-line drugs in symptomless elderly patients.

We prefer to use ACE inhibitors as add-in drugs in patients whose blood pressures are not controlled with either thiazide diuretics or calcium-channel blockers. We also employ ACE inhibitors in patients with diabetes mellitus and heart failure.

In elderly patients where more than one drug is needed to control blood pressure we recommend the combinations as described in Chapter 12. With double therapy there are less striking age-related differences in blood pressure response.

Our aim is to reduce blood pressure in elderly patients to below 150/90 mmHg. It is important for doctors, nurses and patients to appreciate that hypertension is largely a problem of elderly people, and if blood pressure is controlled almost all hypertension-related strokes can be prevented. Now that the benefits of treatment have been confirmed, the next priority is to ensure that all elderly people are screened for hypertension and that all those with raised blood pressure are given the appropriate treatment.

Diabetes mellitus

NIDDM, like hypertension, becomes commoner with advancing age. Such patients need careful dietary counselling as they should be particularly responsive to salt restriction. Where hypertension and diabetes coincide, ACE inhibitors are probably the best first-line drugs because of their reno-protective effects (see Chapter 14). However, because of the associated renin suppression that develops with advancing age and is common in patients with NIDDM, ACE inhibitors (like beta-blockers) tend to be less effective at lowering blood pressure. It is our policy, therefore, to add in a calcium-channel blocker (either amlodipine or slow-release verapamil) rather than increase the dose of the first-line agent. Thiazide diuretics are best avoided in elderly patients with hypertension and NIDDM as they may further impair insulin sensitivity.

Cholesterol

There is insufficient information on the hazards of raised blood cholesterol levels in patients over the age of 70, and the value of cholesterol-lowering drugs has not yet been investigated. Raised blood cholesterol levels become more frequent with advancing age so this is a common problem in elderly hypertensive patients. It is our policy to take a similar line as in non-elderly patients (see Chapter 14).

Elderly patients with coronary artery disease (heart attack or angina pectoris) should receive a statin if their cholesterol levels exceed 5.0 mmol/l. We take a similar threshold in patients who have a history of stroke, transient cerebral ischaemic attack or peripheral vascular disease. In patients who have no evidence of vascular complications of hypertension there is considerable uncertainty, especially in older people. We would definitely prescribe a statin for patients with serum cholesterol levels that are consistently greater than 7.5 mmo/l. The decision on what to do in patients with cholesterol levels between 5.0 and 7.5 mmol/l must depend on concomitant risk factors and their severity. The presence of NIDDM would lower our threshold to around 6.0 mmol/l. Expert dietetic advice should be sought with a comprehensive package of well thought out suggestions on how to correct obesity, maintain a low-fat diet and reduce salt consumption.

FURTHER READING

Avanzini F, Alli C, Bettelli G, et al. Antihypertensive efficacy and tolerability of different drug regimes in isolated systolic hypertension in the elderly. Eur Heart J 1994; **2**: 206–12.

Beard K, Bulpitt CJ, Mascie-Taylor H, et al. Management of elderly patients with sustained hypertension. Br Med J 1992; **304**: 412–6.

Bulpitt CJ, Fletcher AE, Amery A, et al. The hypertension in the very elderly trial (HYVET). J Hum Hypertens 1994; **6**: 631–2.

MRC Working Party. Medical Research Council trial of treatment of hypertension in older adults. Br Med J 1992; **304**: 405–12.

Potter JF. Hypertension in the elderly. Br Med Bull 1994; **50**: 408–19.

SHEP Cooperative Research Group. Prevention of stroke by antihypertensive drug treatment in older person with isolated systolic hypertension. Final results of the Systolic Hypertension in the Elderly Program (SHEP). JAMA 1991; **265**: 3255–64.

Staessen JA, Fagard R, Thijs L, et al for the Systolic Hypertension in Europe (Syst-Eur) Trial Investigators. Randomised double blind comparison of placebo and active treatment for older adults with isolated systolic hypertension. Lancet 1997; **350**: 757–64.

16　HYPERTENSION IN PREGNANCY

BACKGROUND

Hypertension in pregnancy remains one of the most mysterious medical conditions facing the clinician. Whilst it is relatively common, medical science has, to date, failed to provide a coherent mechanism and clinical research has provided only a limited amount of information to guide the clinician when managing individual patients. There are clearly several quite distinct forms of hypertension in pregnancy and they differ not only in terms of pathogenesis but also in terms of treatment. In England and Wales, hypertension ranks equally with pulmonary embolus as the commonest cause of maternal death, with a rate of 10 per million pregnancies. It is also the commonest cause of fetal and neonatal death.

The relative paucity of therapeutic trial data on which to make clinical decisions means that on some occasions obstetricians and physicians have tended to base their opinions on extrapolations from published data concerning older non-pregnant women or even men. There is every reason to believe that this is dangerous and can lead to the mother and baby being exposed to antihypertensive drugs that are at times useless and may even be harmful.

There are some disturbing data on the use of some beta-blockers and the ACE inhibitors in pregnancy. The decision to use these drugs is all too often made on the basis of an inadequate understanding of the mechanism of the hypertensive syndromes of pregnancy, and a failure to respond to advances in our knowledge of the hazards of treatment as well as the benefits.

CLASSIFICATION OF THE HYPERTENSIVE SYNDROMES IN PREGNANCY

There have been several attempts to classify the hypertensive syndromes in pregnancy. None are entirely satisfactory but it is important to attempt to ascertain which syndrome is present in individual patients so that appropriate treatment can be given. In 1997, an extremely useful analysis was published by Brown and Buddle from Australia. The authors took the view that the syndrome of so-called pregnancy-induced hypertension (PIH) was more

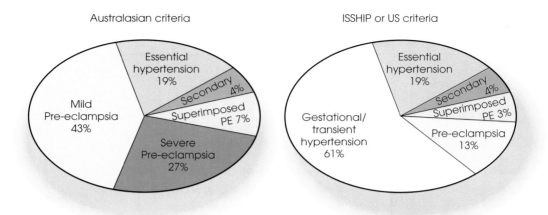

Figure 16.1

A comparison of two classifications of the hypertensive syndromes of pregnancy in 1183 consecutive pregnancies. (*J Hypertens* 1997; **15**: 1049–54.)

likely to be a very mild variant of pre-eclampsia that was not associated with proteinuria. They therefore reviewed the diagnostic classification in 1183 consecutive hypertensive pregnancies according to their new criteria in comparison with the older criteria of the International Society for the Study of Hypertension in Pregnancy (ISSHIP). The results of this analysis are shown in Figure 16.1 and they provide an accurate estimate of the frequency of the various hypertensive syndromes that can be expected in a largely Caucasian population. It is possible that a different picture would be seen in South Asian or African-origin patients where pre-eclampsia may be more common.

Hypertension remains a rare but important cause of maternal death, usually in older women with a poor previous medical or

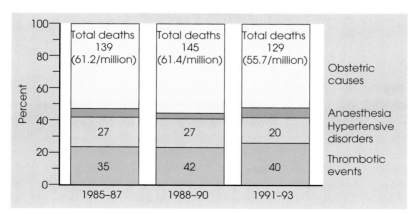

Figure 16.2

Causes of maternal mortality in England and Wales. (Hypertensive maternal mortality approx. 8 deaths per year).

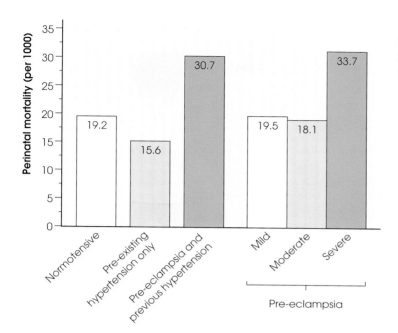

Figure 16.3
Perinatal mortality in relation to blood pressure in the British Births Survey.

obstetrical history. Between 1985 and 1993, 74 women died in Britain as a result of the various hypertensive syndromes of pregnancy (Fig. 16.2).

Pre-existing essential hypertension

About 5% of women of childbearing age have chronic pre-existing, usually mild, essential hypertension, as defined by the World Health Organization criteria, of a blood pressure of 140/90 mmHg or more. In women in their late thirties and early forties, this figure approaches 10%. When these women become pregnant, blood pressure frequently settles during the first trimester but may rise to pre-pregnant levels during the third trimester. Unfortunately, pre-pregnant blood pressure measurements are frequently not available to the clinician, so it is difficult to be certain whether a blood pressure rise in mid-to-late pregnancy is due to early pre-eclampsia, to pregnancy-induced hypertension or to pre-existing mild hypertension.

It is important to note that mild essential hypertension in pregnancy does not carry a bad prognosis for mother or fetus and its early treatment does not convincingly prevent the onset of pre-eclampsia or protect the mother or the baby (Fig. 16.3).

Secondary hypertension in pregnancy

The topic of secondary hypertension is covered in other chapters of this book. Primary hyperaldosteronism is very rare and there is little information available on its management in pregnancy. If present, there will be hypokalaemia and a high or high/normal plasma sodium level. Phaeochromocytomas are well described in pregnancy and are associated with both maternal and fetal death. Hypertension associated with renal disease may cause renal impairment, in which case the patient may be sub-fertile. When pregnancy does occur, the outcome is bad as uraemia has direct effects on the fetus and, furthermore, there may be a non-reversible deterioration of renal function during the pregnancy. Fortunately, this problem is rare in routine clinical practice and such patients need urgent specialist referral.

Diabetes, hypertension and pregnancy

Women of childbearing age may have IDDM or NIDDM. A proportion of these patients will have hypertension. Obese women have a greater risk of both gestational diabetes and raised blood pressure in pregnancy.

Pregnancy-induced hypertension (PIH)

This term refers to those women whose blood pressures are documented to be normal both before and after pregnancy, who sustain a rise in blood pressures in late pregnancy, but who do not develop pre-eclampsia. There are varying criteria for diagnosing PIH and none are entirely satisfactory. The International Society for the Study of Hypertension in Pregnancy defined PIH as a single diastolic blood pressure (phase 5) of 110 mmHg or more or two readings of 90 mmHg or more at least 4 hours apart occurring after the 20th week of pregnancy in a previously normotensive woman. An American Working Group

defines it as a rise of more than 15 mmHg diastolic or 30 mmHg systolic compared with readings taken in early pregnancy. If PIH is mild and does not proceed to pre-eclampsia, then the prognosis is good. It develops in up to 25% of women in their first pregnancy and in 10% of subsequent pregnancies. It is probable that PIH is simply a mild form of pre-eclampsia, which carries a good prognosis.

Pre-eclampsia

This syndrome compared with all others carries a bad prognosis and requires careful assessment and treatment. Pre-eclampsia is diagnosed if the mother develops proteinuria (more than 300 mg/l) associated with a blood pressure that rises to above 140/90 mmHg after the 20th week of pregnancy. The third feature of pre-eclampsia, namely oedema, is much less reliable as mild pre-tibial and facial oedema is common in entirely normal pregnancies. The prevalence of pre-eclampsia is 4–5% in mothers during their first pregnancy and about half this figure in later pregnancies if the father is the same.

Eclampsia

Eclampsia is a major obstetrical emergency associated with a high incidence of both maternal and infant mortality. Blood pressures are almost invariably high and proteinuria of more than 300 mg/l (i.e. dipstick proteinuria one plus or more) is almost always present. There may be gross facial and peripheral oedema, headaches, irritability and, in extreme cases, convulsions. In addition, there may be cerebral and pulmonary oedema, renal failure, hepatic failure, retinal haemorrhages and exudates, retinal detachment and strokes. This terrifying syndrome occurs in around one pregnancy in 500 in the developed world but is commoner in countries that lack efficient antenatal care.

HELLP Syndrome

This syndrome occurs in severe pre-eclampsia and eclampsia is characterised by haemolysis (H), elevated liver enzymes (EL) and low platelets counts (LP). It is associated with a very high maternal and fetal mortality.

DIAGNOSIS

Some of the diagnostic categories above are open to variations in criteria or guidelines laid down by various expert committees and there is often an overlap. Some of the diagnoses can only be made with confidence in retrospect once the pregnancy is over and the mother is assessed 3 months later.

The presence of proteinuria is critical to the diagnosis of pre-eclampsia or eclampsia. The accurate measurement of blood pressure is also of paramount importance, but this topic is sadly neglected.

BLOOD PRESSURE MEASUREMENT IN PREGNANCY

The first recorded measurement of blood pressure in pregnancy was by Frederick Henry Horatio Akbar Mahommed in 1874 at the London Fever Hospital. The invention of the mercury sphygmomanometer by Riva Rocci in 1896 and the discovery of the Korotkov sounds in 1905 meant that the measurement of blood pressure in clinical practice was relatively easy. Sadly, however, standardisation of methods, equipment and the posture of the patient for optimum assessment has not been achieved.

The topic of blood pressure measurement is covered in detail in Chapter 6. In pregnancy, the main sources of variation are the methods for measuring the diastolic pressure and the posture of the patients.

Measurement of diastolic blood pressure

In the past, obstetricians, along with all other clinicians, have tended to take the diastolic blood pressure at the phase of muffling of diastolic sounds (phase 4) rather than the phase of disappearance of sounds (phase 5). This has lead to considerable confusion and still remains the source of some debate. It was argued that in the hyperdynamic state that occurs in pregnancy, faint diastolic sounds are often heard at very low pressure levels, or even at 0 mmHg. It was recommended, therefore, that it would be better to measure the diastolic pressure at the phase of muffling (phase 4). However, intra-arterial blood pressure measurement has clearly demonstrated that the true intra-arterial diastolic pressure is closer to the phase of final disappearance of sounds (phase 5).

More recently, it has been shown that the tendency for phase 5 diastolic pressures to be improbably low was somewhat overestimated (Fig. 16.4). The median difference between the muffling and disappearance phases (i.e. phase 4 minus phase 5) in pregnancy was 2.7 mmHg, whilst in non-pregnant women it was 0.7 mmHg.

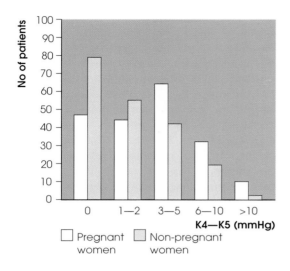

Figure 16.4

The difference between muffling and disappearance of sounds when measuring diastolic blood pressures (K4 minus K5 in mmHg).

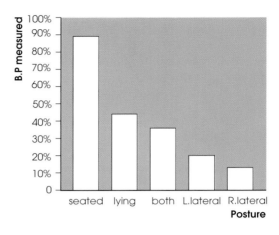

Figure 16.5

Posture favoured by midwives and obstetricians when measuring blood pressure, demonstrating lack of agreement as to the best method.

Furthermore, a recent survey amongst obstetricians and midwives demonstrated that almost half favoured phase 5 and half favoured phase 4 so there is clearly diagnostic anarchy.

Analysis of the techniques reported in the international obstetric literature shows, however, an increasing trend to adopt phase 5. We strongly advocate the universal use of phase 5 for recording diastolic pressure, with the caveat that phase 4 should be used if the K4–K5 difference exceeds 20 mmHg.

Posture

As in the non-pregnant state, we recommend the routine measurement of blood pressure in the seated position (Fig. 16.5). In late pregnancy, when women lie flat on their backs, the gravid uterus may cause some vena caval compression, leading to a reduction of venous return, a fall in cardiac output and a fall in blood pressure; when the patient lies on her side, blood pressure rises. This assessment of blood pressure by the 'roll over test' is now obsolete and provides no useful information.

Routine blood pressure monitoring

Blood pressure should be measured at least monthly for the first two trimesters and thereafter weekly. If the pressure is 140/90 mmHg or more it should be re-measured after 5

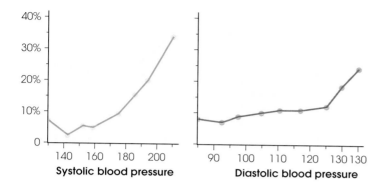

Figure 16.6
Perinatal mortality in relation to systolic and diastolic blood pressure in 4404 women with pre–eclampsia.

minutes' rest in the seated position in a quiet room. If this second blood pressure measurement exceeds 140/90 mm Hg at any stage of pregnancy, accurate clinical assessment of the patient is crucial, and if the pressure exceeds 160/110 mmHg, this should be done on an inpatient basis in most cases.

PROGNOSIS

The prognosis for the various hypertensive syndromes in pregnancy varies according to category. There are only a limited number of reports of perinatal or maternal mortality in relation to accurate assessments of blood pressure in the three trimesters of pregnancy. This is partly because, in developed countries, maternal and perinatal mortality is so low that risk factors have to be investigated using national surveillance statistics and these data tend to rely on casual and often inaccurate blood pressure measurement by thousands of observers.

Very high blood pressure in pregnancy can affect the mother and the baby. In the mother, there is an increased risk of pre-eclampsia, but also an increased risk of stroke and renal damage. The consequences to the fetus are reduced uteroplacental blood flow, placental ischaemia, intra-uterine growth retardation, premature delivery, abruptio placentae (ante partum haemorrhage) and fetal death (Fig. 16.6).

National surveillance data demonstrate that the perinatal mortality in pregnancies associated with mild essential hypertension and mild PIH is, in fact, somewhat lower than in the majority of pregnancies where the blood pressure remains persistently normal. By sharp contrast, there is a high perinatal mortality in those pregnancies complicated by proteinuric pre-eclampsia. The reasons for the good outlook in the mild hypertensive woman with no pre-eclampsia are uncertain. It may be because those mothers who were diagnosed as having mildly raised blood pressure received a higher quality of obstetrical care. Alternatively, the mothers with lower blood pressure included a sub-group who had other diseases, like asthma or chronic infections, which may have reduced their blood pressures.

Whatever the mechanisms of the lack of adverse effects of mild hypertension alone, there are important clinical implications. Mild hypertension with blood pressures below 150/100 mm Hg in pregnancy should not be treated with antihypertensive drugs. Clearly, careful observation is crucial as in some cases blood pressures may rise to levels where drug therapy is necessary and the clinician is not able to predict whose pressures will rise and whose will not.

There is no convincing evidence that the treatment of mild hypertension in pregnancy has any effect in preventing pre-eclampsia, or reducing the incidence of intra-uterine growth retardation or preterm delivery.

AETIOLOGY

Hypertension in pregnancy has been called the 'disease of theories', mainly because a great many hypotheses have been advanced but none convincingly fit the bill. Clues may be obtained from investigating the epidemiology of pre-eclampsia and from studies of its pathology.

Epidemiology of hypertension in pregnancy

Large-scale studies have demonstrated that certain mothers are particularly prone to developing pre-eclampsia. Their identification can aid in their management.

Genetic factors

Pre-eclampsia undoubtedly runs in families and is likely to be due to genetic factors as well as a tendency for relatives to be subjected to similar environmental influences.

An autosomal dominant inheritance has been postulated by some researchers but this may only operate in a minority of cases.

Age

There is an increased incidence of pre-eclampsia in young teenage girls and in women aged over 35 years.

Parity

Pre-eclampsia is commonest in first pregnancies and in women with five or more pregnancies, with a rate of about 6%. The syndrome is more common in second or third pregnancies if they are by a different father. With both first and second fathers, the risk of pre-eclampsia is inversely related to the duration of sexual cohabitation prior to conception.

Multiple pregnancies

Pregnancies associated with both monozygotic and dizygotic twins have a raised rate of pre-eclampsia.

Previous pre-eclampsia

Mothers who have had pre-eclampsia in their first pregnancy have an increased chance of this developing in subsequent pregnancies, although the risk is low.

Previous oral contraceptive-induced hypertension

It is generally held that women who have had raised blood pressure on oral contraceptives have an increased risk of hypertension in pregnancy. It is uncertain whether this is true for the newer low-oestrogen or progestagen-only contraceptive. Similarly, there is some doubt whether women who develop hypertension in pregnancy have a greater chance of developing raised blood pressure if they subsequently use oral contraceptives.

Ethnic origin

Pre-eclampsia is commoner in black and Asian people in the UK, but it is uncertain whether this is due to environmental and social factors or to any genuine ethnic difference.

Obesity

Maternal obesity is associated with pre-eclampsia as well as a greater tendency to develop essential hypertension. If appropriate sized arm cuffs are used in blood pressure measurement, the effects of obesity are less pronounced. It is uncertain whether women who gain more weight during pregnancy are at greater risk of pre-eclampsia.

Socio-economic factors

People of low socio-economic status are more prone to most diseases and this is true for hypertension in general as well as for hypertension in pregnancy. Assuming only a modest genetic determinant of pre-eclampsia, then the socio-economic gradient is likely to be related to obesity, poor quality diet and overcrowding. Paradoxically, cigarette smoking does not cause pre-eclampsia, nor does it cause hypertension in non-pregnant people. Cigarette smoking does, however, cause fetal growth retardation.

Other factors

Pre-eclampsia is commoner in diabetic women, those with hydatidiform mole and Rhesus iso-immunisation. Pregnancies leading to male babies have a slightly higher risk of eclampsia.

Pathogenesis

Pre-eclampsia appears to be a syndrome associated with a defect of implantation of the placenta, and thus has its origins in early pregnancy, before any clinical features are detectable. At this early stage, there is histological evidence of a reduced number of uteroplacental arteries and a failure of the spiral arteries, in particular, to dilate, lose their muscularis, and thus provide for an increase in blood flow that will become necessary later on in pregnancy as the fetus grows. The placenta and fetus are thus ischaemic at an early stage. Subsequently, the development of atherosis, fibroblastic proliferation and fibrinoid necrosis causes more acute ischaemia with vascular occlusions and placental infarctions. Non-infarcted areas of the placenta look pale and gritty. The fetus is ischaemic and hypoxic, growth is retarded and, in severe cases, the fetus dies. Renal involvement, with the development of proteinuria and elevation of blood pressure, are late phenomena and should be regarded as secondary to the basic underlying disease of the placenta.

MECHANISMS

The search for the mechanisms of pre-eclampsia has centred on investigations of vaso-active substances and intravascular clotting factors. As with similar studies in non-pregnant hypertensive women, it is often difficult to be certain whether the findings are a cause or a consequence of the raised blood pressure.

The renin-angiotensin system

Renin is generated by the kidney, but there is also good evidence that there are local renin–angiotensin systems in the placenta and uterus. Thus, circulating renin and angiotensin levels may not reflect the true role of the renin system in pregnancy. In normal pregnancy, plasma renin substrate (angiotensinogen) levels are high, and renin is consumed to generate angiotensin II so that plasma renin activity is raised. In hypertensive pregnancies, these trends are less pronounced and plasma renin activity is lower, but still not as low as in the non-pregnant state. Thus, in normal pregnancies the circulating renin–angiotensin system is activated, and in hypertensive pregnancies it is less active. The lower levels of angiotensin II may be related to increased vascular sensitivity to endogenous and exogenous (infused) angiotensin II.

The local renin–angiotensin systems have received less attention, but may promote vasoconstriction, vessel wall growth and failure of dilatation of the spiral arteries. Angiotensin may exert some positive effects on fetal growth and development.

Women with severe pre-eclampsia or eclampsia may develop a clinical condition not unlike the malignant phase of hypertension, with fibrinoid necrosis of their intra-renal arterioles. This leads to juxtaglomerular ischaemia and the production of large quantities of renin and high circulating levels of angiotensin II.

Other vaso-active substances

There is evidence of disturbance of function of many vaso-active systems in pre-eclampsia. These include increased vascular responsiveness to adrenaline and noradrenaline, reductions in vasodilator prostaglandin production, and low levels of kallikrein–kinin activity; also, a possible role for the newly discovered vasoconstrictor, endothelin, has been suggested. These abnormalities are clearly all inter-related and their individual significance is uncertain.

Coagulation

A certain degree of activation of the coagulation system, with thrombin-mediated fibrin generation, is a feature of normal pregnancy. In pre-eclampsia, fibrinolytic activity may be impaired and platelet aggregation is increased. In extreme cases, a consumptive coagulopathy develops with thrombocytopenia, micro-angiopathic haemolytic anaemia, a rise in circulating fibrin degradation products and a prolonged prothrombin time. Measurement of these features is used in monitoring the clinical management of moderate-to-severe pre-eclamptic mothers.

Haemodynamics

In a normal pregnancy, there is a rise in plasma volume and cardiac output and a fall in total peripheral resistance. There is a slight tendency of blood pressure to fall in the first half of a normal pregnancy. In mothers with pre-eclampsia, cardiac output is reduced, plasma volume falls and peripheral resistance rises. Resistance to blood flow in the uteroplacental circulation increases and this further compounds the tendency to fetoplacental ischaemia.

CLINICAL MANAGEMENT

As outlined above, accurate blood pressure measurement is essential because even small elevations of pressure do radically affect the patient's care. Similarly, patients need very careful general assessment to check for underlying causes of hypertension and to detect other clinical conditions that may influence the choice of antihypertensive drugs.

Hypertension before pregnancy

It is now generally agreed that it is the responsibility of the primary health care team to ensure that all adults have their blood pressures measured regularly. This has led to an increasing number of women of childbearing age being diagnosed as having hypertension. Clearly, decisions on what to do depend on the degree of elevation of the blood pressure and whether it is associated with underlying renal or adrenal disease. It should be remembered, however, that relatively young pre-menopausal women do not have a high hypertension-related, absolute cardiovascular risk; i.e. their actual chance of developing a heart attack or a stroke is minimal, particularly if

they are non-smokers with a benign family history. The clinician is faced with the question as to whether drug therapy should be started. The British Hypertension Society guidelines for the management of hypertension also give the clinician a mandate to withhold drug therapy in very low-risk, very mild hypertensives. Many women of childbearing potential fall into this category, although they must be monitored regularly.

If the clinician does opt to prescribe antihypertensive drugs then he or she must bear in mind that the patient may at some time become pregnant. There should be a natural reluctance to prescribe any drugs in 'potentially pregnant' women. In particular, the clinician should remember that ACE inhibitors are absolutely contraindicated in pregnancy as they are associated with a high perinatal mortality. The calcium-channel blockers are relatively contraindicated, diuretics should not be used in pregnancy and some (but not all) beta-blockers are associated with adverse fetal outcome.

The assessment of hypertensive patients who are not pregnant is covered in Chapters 7 and 8, and in young women special efforts must be made to detect underlying causes.

There are very few women who should be advised to avoid becoming pregnant on account of their hypertension. With modern antihypertensive drugs, the risk of stroke in pregnancy can be greatly reduced. If women with severe hypertension do become pregnant, then early expert obstetrical and medical care is necessary.

Hypertension before 20 weeks of gestation

If women are found to have blood pressures of 140/90 mmHg or more at the first antenatal visit, they should preferably

Table 16.1

The results of a trial with labetolol or methyldopa or no therapy in mild hypertension in early pregnancy.

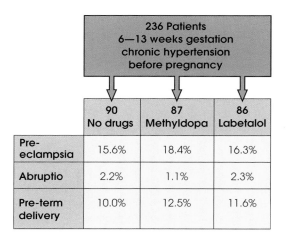

	90 No drugs	87 Methyldopa	86 Labetalol
Pre-eclampsia	15.6%	18.4%	16.3%
Abruptio	2.2%	1.1%	2.3%
Pre-term delivery	10.0%	12.5%	11.6%

be referred to a joint antenatal–hypertension clinic. It is probable that hypertension at this stage is really due to underlying chronic, essential or secondary hypertension, especially if obesity is present. A strong family history of hypertension would certainly suggest that the patient has essential hypertension.

All such patients should undergo routine dipstick urine testing and a blood sample should be taken for a haematological profile and serum levels of urea, creatinine, uric acid, sodium and potassium as well as a random blood glucose. A 24-hour urine test for catecholamine excretion should also be started. If the blood pressure exceeds 160/110 mmHg, then it may be preferable to admit the patient to the antenatal ward for more detailed assessment. If the blood pressure remains at this level, antihypertensive medication should be started, usually with labetalol or methyldopa. The choice of antihypertensive drugs is described later in this chapter.

The use of antihypertensive drugs in the treatment of mild hypertensive women in early pregnancy has not been shown to be useful (Table 16.1). One study employing atenolol provided worrying results, as the fetuses subjected to atenolol rather than placebo were 1 kg lighter (Table 16.2). If, therefore, blood pressure remains at 150/100 mmHg or less, antihypertensive drugs should not be prescribed.

Table 16.2

The results of a randomised trial of atenolol versus placebo in mild hypertension in early pregnancy.

	Gestation at entry (weeks)	BP at entry (mmHg K5)	In-trial BP (mmHg K5)	Birth weight (kg)	Placental weight (g)	Weight at 1 year (kg)
Atenolol (n = 15)	15.8	144/86	132/74	2.62	454	9.26
Placebo (n = 14)	15.9	148/86	136/81	3.53	633	9.82

If both hypertension and proteinuria are present before 20 weeks of gestation, then it is likely that there is some underlying renal pathology such as glomerulonephritis or pyelonephritis. Bacteriological examination of the urine is essential and, where relevant, antibiotic drugs should be given. If the serum creatinine exceeds 100 mmol/l the kidneys should be imaged by ultrasonography.

Hypertension after 20 weeks of gestation

Elevation of blood pressure for the first time after 20 weeks of gestation is likely to be due to PIH or, if proteinuria also develops, the mother may have pre-eclampsia. The clinical problem is that the clinician may not be sure which of these two symptoms is developing.

Pregnancy-induced hypertension

If there is a modest blood pressure rise in the second half of pregnancy and this is not associated with proteinuria or severe oedema, then the outlook is good. If the pressure exceeds 160/110 mm Hg, then admission to hospital and antihypertensive medication are recommended. If the pressures are between 140/90 and 160/110 mm Hg, then many women can be managed at home, with rest — but not bed rest. Those who are still at work should stop. The midwives or obstetricians should check blood pressure at least twice weekly. If it remains above 150/100 mm Hg, and there is no proteinuria, then most clinicians would start antihypertensive medication on an outpatient basis. The limited number of clinical trials on the use of beta-blockers, labetalol and methyldopa suggest no adverse outcome when treating this level of blood pressure in late pregnancy, but there was no evidence of prevention of pre-eclampsia. This level of pressure is associated with an appreciable risk of stroke, particularly in high-risk, older mothers. The risk is, however, too small for any single clinical trial to have the power to detect a difference between placebo or active drug therapy.

Pre-eclampsia

This syndrome is serious and is associated with intra-uterine growth retardation or death, as well as maternal morbidity and mortality. If blood pressure rises after 20 weeks of gestation, and proteinuria develops, the mother should be admitted to hospital immediately for full assessment and antihypertensive medication. Whilst strict bed rest is of no value (and may be harmful), the simple process of admitting the patient may cause a fall in blood pressure.

The clinical progress should be monitored with 4-hourly blood pressure readings, twice-weekly measurements of serum creatinine and uric acid levels and platelet counts, as well as twice-weekly 24-hour urine collections for protein estimations.

If pre-eclampsia develops very near to the end of the pregnancy, then the optimum treatment is to deliver the baby whilst maintaining good blood pressure control until 7 days post partum. Mothers should also be prescribed diazepam or phenytoin as well as magnesium sulphate to prevent eclamptic convulsions. Severely pre-eclamptic patients who have blood pressures over 160/110 mm Hg and show signs of cerebral irritability or headaches should be admitted to an intensive care unit. Furthermore, if the pregnancy is not far advanced (i.e. less than 35 weeks), the mother should be admitted to a hospital with excellent paediatric back-up with a special care baby unit. Such units can almost guarantee the survival of fetuses weighing as little as 1 kg.

Eclampsia

With improvements in antenatal care, this syndrome should become increasingly uncommon. The mother's life is in great danger. In addition to anticonvulsant drugs, blood pressure should be reduced with parenteral medication with labetalol miniboluses (50 mg) or infusions of intravenous hydralazine (20 mg). Magnesium sulphate is now regarded as the best anticonvulsant and also has some antihypertensive properties. In milder cases, control of blood pressure can be achieved with oral nifedipine (not slow release). However, precipitate drops in pressure should be avoided as this can worsen cerebral, cardiac, renal and placental ischaemia.

The management of full-blown eclampsia is the responsibility of the obstetrician, together with an anaesthetist and a paediatrician, and is covered in more detail in obstetrical textbooks.

INVESTIGATIONS

Renal function

Serum urea and creatinine levels should be measured in all mothers at the first antenatal booking and again if the blood pressure rises. A serum urea of more than 5 mmol/l and a serum creatinine of 100 mmol/l or more are highly abnormal in a pregnant woman and suggest a diagnosis of renal impairment.

Electrolytes

Plasma potassium may be reduced due to high-dose diuretic therapy, which should not be prescribed in pregnancy anyway. In primary aldosteronism, serum potassium is low and serum sodium is moderately elevated.

In severe pre-eclampsia, serum sodium and potassium may fall to low levels due to intense hyperaldosteronism induced by renal ischaemia and hepatic dysfunction.

Uric acid

Serum uric acid levels are sometimes modestly raised in patients with essential hypertension, so this test should be done, at first booking, in all hypertensive mothers. In pre-eclampsia, hyperuricaemia frequently develops, and this may be used to confirm the diagnosis and monitor progress. The value of serial measurements of serum uric acid levels is debatable as they tend only to become abnormal in clinically obvious pre-eclampsia.

Haematological indices

In severe pre-eclampsia and eclampsia, there is a consumptive coagulopathy that is associated with thrombocytopenia, a prolonged prothrombin time (or raised INR) and increased fibrin degradation products and plasma levels of fibrin D-dimer. These parameters should be monitored regularly. If coagulopathy is present, the outlook is bad, and emergency lower segment caesarian section should be considered.

Ultrasound scans

Fetal progress should be monitored throughout pregnancy by serial measurements of crown-rump length (CRL) by ultrasound. In later pregnancy, fetal growth is monitored by serial measurements of biparietal diameter

(BPD). This is the best method of diagnosing intra-uterine growth retardation.

Cardiotocograph

Once the pregnancy has advanced beyond 20 weeks, patients can be monitored by cardiotocography (CTG). This should demonstrate physiological beat-to-beat variation of fetal heart rate and the response when the baby kicks or there is a spontaneous uterine contraction. If there is fetal distress, there is a loss of variability of heart rate and also sudden decelerations. As with all antenatal monitoring, this test has a high level of specificity (i.e. few false positives) but low sensitivity (i.e. many false negatives).

Proteinuria

The detection of proteinuria is crucial to obstetrical care and, when it is present, protein 24-hour urine excretion should be measured. At the present state of knowledge, the measurement of microproteinuria as a method of diagnosing early pre-eclampsia cannot be recommended.

ANTIHYPERTENSIVE REGIMES

The information available on the safety of antihypertensive drugs in pregnancy is very limited and with the newer agents like the ACE inhibitors and the calcium-channel blockers there are so few published data that these drugs should be avoided. It should be noted that the manufacturers of these drugs specifically state that they are contraindicated in pregnancy. The clinician should, therefore, be very conservative in the choice of drugs and should think hard before prescribing anything.

Rest and sedation

Bed rest is of no value. With rest blood pressure settles but, as soon as the patient mobilises again, the pressure rises and nothing has been achieved. There is no published evidence that bed rest leads to a favourable outcome in pregnancy, and it may lead to an increased risk of venous thrombosis or pulmonary embolus. A less strict form of rest, by stopping work and 'taking things easy' at home or in the ward can, however, be advised, although its blood pressure-lowering effects are not impressive.

Sedatives and tranquillisers are similarly of no value unless the patient is agitated or distressed. These drugs may sometimes produce an uncontrolled and prolonged fall in blood pressure, and may cause hypotonia and hypothermia in the fetus. The technique of treating hypertension in pregnancy with bed rest and sedatives represents archaic obstetrical practice, which is known to be useless.

Diazepam may, however, be used as an alternative to phenytoin in patients with eclampsia or severe pre-eclampsia as they have a high risk of developing convulsions.

Salt restriction

There is little information on the value of salt restriction in pregnancy. Extreme salt restriction may reduce intravascular volume and stimulate renin release, so it is best avoided. It seems sensible to suggest a maximum sodium intake of around 100 mmol/day, this being about two-thirds of the average intake in northern European and American populations. This salt intake is easily achievable by not adding salt at the table or in cooking and restricting notoriously salty foods like hamburgers, sausages and salted snacks.

Weight restriction

Rigorous dieting should be avoided in pregnancy, although obese patients should be advised to try to avoid excessive weight gain in pregnancy and to moderate their calorie intake.

Antihypertensive drugs

A comprehensive review of antihypertensive drugs is to be found in Chapter 11. The review here concentrates on the use of drugs in pregnancy, although the other aspects of each pharmacological group should be borne in mind.

Diuretics

The thiazides are said to be contraindicated in pregnancy. Women with pre-eclampsia have relatively contracted plasma volumes and diuretics will cause further reduction and worsen the impairment of uteroplacental blood flow. However, a recent review has suggested that diuretics are not as harmful as they were originally thought to be. Diuretics, particularly frusemide, may, of course, prove necessary if there is severe heart failure or gross fluid retention due to renal failure.

Centrally acting drugs

Methyldopa has, for many years, been the mainstay of obstetrical antihypertensive treatment. There is good evidence that it is entirely safe in pregnancy for both mother and baby, but the drug is now falling from favour because it causes severe dose-related sedation and lethargy. Methyldopa probably does remain the first-line drug in women with asthma, where beta-blockers are contraindicated. Doses of up to 2 g daily can be used, but sedation can be minimised with no more than 750 mg daily.

In theory, the use of methyldopa in pregnancy might be associated with the development of postnatal depression, although there are no reliable reports of this.

Labetalol

This drug has been used extensively in pregnancy and there is no evidence of any adverse effects. The starting dose is usually 100 mg twice daily, doubling if necessary. If, with a total of 400 mg daily, blood pressure remains uncontrolled, then it is usual to add in either hydralazine or nifedipine.

Beta-blockers

Published data on the use of beta-blockers that lack intrinsic sympathomimetic activity (ISA) are alarming, with reduced fetal blood flow and smaller babies. Drugs like atenolol and propranolol should now be regarded as contraindicated in pregnancy. Oxprenolol and pindolol, both of which have ISA, may be safe but are not used much nowadays.

Hydralazine

When given by injection, hydralazine is useful in the treatment of severe pre-eclampsia and eclampsia. Its use in the milder grades of hypertension has declined as newer drugs have become available. Oral hydralazine is a safe alternative to beta-blockers or methyldopa in the earlier stages of pregnancy.

Calcium-channel blockers

There is too little information on the use of calcium-channel blockers in pregnancy to justify their use, except in special circumstances. Nifedipine has been used safely in some severely hypertensive women, either as add-on therapy or where other drugs were contraindicated or not tolerated.

ACE inhibitors

These agents are absolutely contraindicated in pregnancy or, for that matter, in women who are planning to become pregnant. Where they have been used, there are reports of congenital abnormalities, growth retardation and intra-uterine death. However, if ACE inhibitors are discontinued in early pregnancy, fetal outcome has been reported to be favourable.

The alpha-blockers

The world experience suggests that prazocin is not harmful, but there are no reliable data on the use of the newer, long-acting alpha-blockers (doxazocin and terazocin) in pregnancy.

Aspirin

There is some evidence, particularly from the CLASP study, that the use of low-dose aspirin is associated with a reduced risk of placental ischaemia and fetal problems in very high risk pregnancies only. However, this treatment must be started early in the second trimester. Women with hypertension alone should not take aspirin unless there are other factors indicating a high obstetrical risk.

POSTNATAL HYPERTENSION

Post-partum pre-eclampsia or eclampsia

Occasionally, women with mild hypertension in pregnancy sustain a sharp rise in blood pressure up to 10 days after delivery. This may rarely be associated with clinical features of pre-eclampsia or even eclampsia with grand mal convulsions. This syndrome develops even when there is a complete evacuation of the placenta and thus is very surprising. Blood pressures should be monitored carefully in the early postnatal phase, and if diastolic pressures exceed 100 mmHg, antihypertensive drug therapy should be continued and if necessary increased.

Antihypertensive drugs

If hypertension is due to pre-eclampsia alone, blood pressure usually returns to normal within a few days after the baby is born. Thus antihypertensive drugs can gradually be withdrawn gradually over 2 or 3 days. However, blood pressure sometimes remain mildly raised for weeks or months following delivery. Usually it is not high enough to merit drug therapy but patients must be monitored carefully. If the raised blood pressure was due to pre-existing hypertension, with or without pre-eclampsia, therapy should be continued, although frequently the dosage of antihypertensive drugs can be reduced. As thiazides are useful antihypertensive drugs when used in combination with beta-blockers, these may be reintroduced.

Further investigation

All women who have had hypertension of any cause in pregnancy should be referred soon after delivery to a blood pressure clinic. In those women who had pure pre-eclampsia, blood pressures usually return to normal and, apart from a careful history and examination, no further action is needed. If blood pressures remain even slightly elevated after 3 months, then a full work-up with renal imaging is necessary. The methods of managing such patients are covered in Chapter 7.

Further pregnancy

Women who have had lone pre-eclampsia can be reassured that a further pregnancy may not be complicated by the same troubles. However, it is important that, as soon as they become pregnant again, they should attend a joint antenatal and blood pressure clinic. Women with pre-existing hypertension can usually be advised that it is safe to undergo a further pregnancy, but only with careful supervision as they do have an increased risk of stillbirth. Perhaps only women with hypertension complicated by chronic renal failure should be advised to desist from further pregnancies.

SPECIAL SITUATIONS

Chronic renal disease

If the mother has pre-existing chronic renal disease, with or without hypertension, special care is necessary. Superadded pre-eclampsia is common, and it is important to measure the 24-hour urinary protein content at an early stage, usually during a brief in-patient stay. Aggressive control of blood pressure is mandatory but, even then, as many as 45% of pregnancies may end with a dead baby. The help of a nephrologist or hypertension specialist should be sought as soon as pregnancy is diagnosed.

Phaeochromocytoma

This is an important but rare cause of maternal as well as fetal death. A 24-hour urine collection for urinary catecholamines should be routine in all hypertensive pregnancies. If phaeochromocytoma is suggested by this test, then abdominal ultrasound should be undertaken to locate the tumour. It is mandatory that the mother is treated with both alpha- and beta-blockers throughout the whole of the pregnancy. Delivery of the baby is best by caesarian section; a surgeon should be present with a highly qualified anaesthetist, as well as a physician and a paediatrician. If all goes smoothly, it is probably best to remove the phaeochromocytoma electively a week or two after delivery, through a more appropriate abdominal incision, and after CT scanning has confirmed the site of the phaeochromocytoma.

Coronary heart disease

Occasionally, hypertensive women with angina become pregnant. Beta-blockers, with or without calcium-channel blockers, and nitrates are mandatory. Vaginal delivery should be avoided, as should excessive blood pressure falls during epidural anaesthesia.

Asthma

This is a common problem. The asthma is treated along conventional lines. Reliance should be placed more on inhaled beta-agonists, steroids and atropine-like drugs than on oral therapy. Beta-blockers should never be used as even the most cardiose-lective blockers increase airways resistance. High blood pressure should be treated with methyldopa, hydralazine or possibly nifedipine.

Diabetes mellitus

Both IDDM and NIDDM are associated with an increased perinatal mortality rate, and there is evidence that rigorous control of blood glucose levels is associated with a more favourable outcome. Hypertension may frequently be present and it is generally considered that this also should be treated aggressively. The ACE inhibitors are frequently used in diabetic hypertensive patients because of their presumed renoprotective effects. However, in pregnancy, these agents are specifically contraindicated. Atenolol, also commonly used in diabetic patients, should probably be replaced by labetalol.

ORAL CONTRACEPTIVES

Women who have had raised blood pressure in pregnancy are not doomed to develop raised blood pressure when taking the oral contraceptive. However, they should be monitored carefully before starting the pill and thereafter every 6 months. Progestagen-only oral contraceptives are the preferred option.

HYPERTENSION IN LATER LIFE

It is probable that women who have had pre-eclampsia are more likely to develop essential hypertension in later life. They should be regarded as a group to be selectively screened for hypertension in primary care at least once a year.

FURTHER READING

Brown MA, Buddle ML. What's in a name? Problems with the classification of hypertension in pregnancy. *J Hypertens* 1997; **15**: 1049–54.

Lip GYH, Churchill D, Beevers M, *et al*. Angiotensin converting enzyme inhibitors in early pregnancy. *Lancet* 1997; **350**: 1446–7.

Lowe S, Rubin PC. The pharmacological management of hypertension in pregnancy. *J Hypertens* 1992; **10:** 201–7.

National High Blood Pressure Education Program Working Group Report on High Blood Pressure in Pregnancy. *Amer J Obstet Gynaecol* 1986; **163:** 1689–712.

Perry IJ, Stewart BA, Brockwell J, et al. Recording diastolic blood pressure in pregnancy. *Br Med J* 1990; **301:** 1198.

Tunbridge RDG. The management of pregnancy in hypertensive patients. *Postgrad Med J* 1994; **70:** 790–7.

17 BLOOD PRESSURE IN CHILDREN

BACKGROUND

From a clinical point of view, the topic of blood pressure in children has been rather neglected, being mainly of interest to paediatric nephrologists. Only a tiny minority of children need antihypertensive drug therapy and most of these have identifiable renal or vascular abnormalities requiring detailed and expert management.

Long-term, follow-up studies of cohorts of normal infants and children strongly suggest, however, that the origins of adult essential hypertension are to be found in early childhood or even in the antenatal period. These studies, which are difficult to conduct, are in a position to provide an insight into aetiology and may also provide guidance for early non-pharmacological management as well as the primary prevention of hypertension.

BLOOD PRESSURE MEASUREMENT

The principles of blood pressure measurement in children are largely the same as in adults, and the reader is referred to Chapter 6. The main differences are related to arm size, which precludes conventional sphygmomanometry below the age of about 5 years and influences the choice of cuff in all children until they have stopped growing.

Doppler ultrasound blood pressure measurement

In neonates and children up to the age of 5 years, the measurement of blood pressure is best performed by Doppler ultrasound equipment. This only provides a measure of the systolic blood pressure but results are reproducible and accurately reflect the intra-arterial systolic pressure. False elevations of blood pressure can be avoided if the child is quiet, relaxed and not crying. Limited availability of equipment means that this technique is only performed in specialised paediatric units. As conventional sphygmomanometers are not suitable in children under the age of 5 years, the routine measurement of blood pressure cannot be recommended in the context of primary health care.

Oscillometric blood pressure measurement

The use of oscillometric systems for measuring blood pressure is feasible in children of

Table 17.1

Cuff sizes for use in children.

Age	Bladder width (cm)	Bladder length (cm)
Newborn	2.5–4.0	5.0–9.0
Infants (6 months to 3 years)	4.0–6.0	11.5–18.0
Children (3 years to 10 years)	7.5–9.0	17.0–19.0
Small adult size	12.5–13.5	22.0–23.5
Alternative adult size	13.5	33.5

all ages (Chapter 6). There are, however, few published reports of their application on a large scale. Oscillometric manometers generally derive the diastolic blood pressure more closely to the fifth phase of Korotkov sounds. However, to date, none of these devices have been formally evaluated in children. Unfortunately, many semi-automatic manometers, when tested in adults, have proved inaccurate.

Cuff sizes

The topic of cuff sizes in all age groups is not yet fully resolved. It is generally recommended that the rubber bladder inside the cuff should encircle at least 80% of the upper arm. If too small a cuff is used, blood pressure will be overestimated. It remains uncertain whether it matters if the cuff is too big, encircling more than 80% or even overlapping around the arm. Ideally, the paediatrician needs a variety of cuffs to allow for different lengths, as well as circumferences, of childrens' arms. The clinician must use the cuffs that are available and this will differ from country to country. In the UK, there are four cuffs suitable for use in children and, of course, in older children the

conventional 'normal adult' cuff may be suitable (Table 17.1). If there is any doubt, the arm circumference should be measured and the most appropriate cuff employed.

Stethoscope

In very small children, a stethoscope with a paediatric size chest piece is necessary. The stethoscope diaphragm may be more suitable than the bell.

Systolic end-point

The height of the systolic blood pressure can be measured either by palpation of the radial artery or by listening over the brachial artery in the conventional manner. Systolic pressure is taken at the first appearance of the Korotkov sounds.

Diastolic end-point

There remains confusion as to whether muffling or disappearance of the Korotkov sounds provides the most accurate or reproducible estimate of the diastolic blood pressure in children. In adult practice, the disappearance of sounds (Korotkov phase 5) is now universally accepted as the correct method for measuring diastolic pressures. Many paediatricians still take diastolic pressures at the phase of muffling of sounds (phase 4), but we know of no evidence as to whether phase 4 is nearer to the true intra-arterial diastolic pressure than phase 5 in children. If diastolic muffling cannot be identified, then the disappearance of sounds must be employed anyway.

Arm position

It is critical that the arm cuff is at the same level as the heart. The posture of the child will depend on its age. Blood pressures are best measured seated, with the child either in a chair or on the mother's lap.

The flush method for measuring blood pressure

This technique is now obsolete. It depends on the use of a tourniquet and occlusion bandages to render the arm bloodless so that the clinician can then identify at what level of systolic pressure blood returns to the arm as the cuff is deflated.

Leg blood pressure

All children with raised blood pressure should be checked to exclude the diagnosis of aortic coarctation. Blood pressure must be measured in the legs. The child is placed lying on its tummy and a suitable cuff is applied around the thigh, to encircle at least 80% of the circumference. The stethoscope is applied in the popliteal fossa and blood pressure is measured in the conventional auscultatory manner.

Number of readings

As in adult medicine, two blood pressure readings should be taken at each consultation, and the second reading used for clinical decision making. In all but a tiny minority of children with very high blood pressures, rechecking is necessary on at least four occasions before long-term therapeutic decisions are made.

BLOOD PRESSURE IN NORMAL CHILDREN

The results of long-term follow-up studies from the UK and USA are summarised in Figure 17.1. In neonates, blood pressure rises sharply soon after birth from around 90/70 mm Hg to 110/80 mm Hg at about 6 weeks of age. Then blood pressures seem to level off until the age of about 5 years, when a slow steady rise in blood pressure with advancing age is seen, and this trend continues on into adult life. It is not known whether breast-fed babies differ with respect to blood pressure when compared with bottle-fed babies, but there is evidence that babies weaned onto a low-salt diet have a smaller rise in blood pressure over 6 months (2 mmHg) compared with normal salt intake babies (Figure 17.2). The role of salt in the rise in blood pressure with age is discussed in detail in Chapter 3. The development of

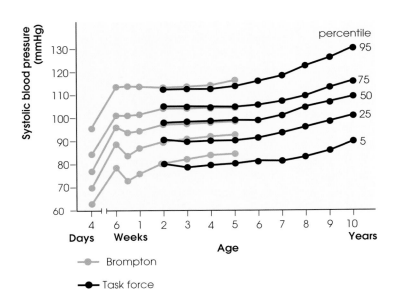

Figure 17.1
Percentiles of systolic blood pressure from the Brompton study and the Task Force for blood pressure control in children.

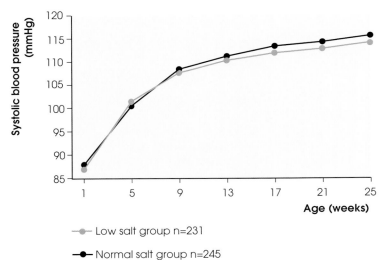

Figure 17.2
A randomised trial of low sodium intake and blood pressure in newborn infants.

essential hypertension is intimately linked to the rise in blood pressure in normal people with advancing age. This phenomenon is not seen in low salt eating societies. Clearly, therefore, the origins of hypertension are to be found in childhood, even in children whose pressures, whilst technically normal, are above average for their age.

Tracking

The term 'tracking' implies that those individuals with blood pressures in the upper, middle or lower parts of the normal range will retain their rank and, as their pressures continue to rise with age, some will cross an arbitrary line and will be considered to have hypertension. Tracking is seen in studies of schoolchildren and young adults, but there is less convincing evidence of tracking of individual pressures in neonates and infants. Thus, it is not possible to predict the onset of clinical hypertension from the blood pressures of neonates and, anyway, a great many other genetic and environmental factors will influence blood pressure over the ensuing decades.

There is also some evidence of a 'vicious cycle effect'. Not only do blood pressures tend to rise with advancing age, but there is evidence, in adults at least, that those individuals with higher pressures sustain a steeper rise than those whose pressures are in the lower part of the distribution. Again, this effect cannot be detected in neonates and infants but is seen in studies of adolescents and young adults.

Genetic factors

Comparison of parents with their adopted and natural children suggests that all children have pressures that positively correlate with those of their parents but that adopted children correlate less closely. Thus, both genetic and shared environmental (mainly dietary) factors are related to the blood pressure of normal children (see Chapter 3).

Birth weight

Recent research has drawn attention to the fact that the birth weight of children is negatively related to blood pressure in adult life. Paradoxically, the low birth weight babies are the ones who develop hypertension in adulthood. As high blood pressure in adults is positively correlated with obesity, this implies that high blood pressure will be seen in individuals who start out being underweight and later become overweight.

The origins of essential hypertension might, therefore, be traced back to the intra-uterine environment and undernutrition, related to poverty and a poor diet, together with later overnutrition, with obesity and an equally poor but different diet. More recently, a close inverse correlation has been demonstrated between maternal blood pressure and birth weight. Higher than average maternal pressures may be harmful to the fetus; and the tendency for these offspring to have higher pressures in later life may simply be due to genetic inheritance.

CRITERIA FOR ABNORMAL BLOOD PRESSURE

As stated in earlier chapters, it is difficult to define normal blood pressure. All blood pressures in Western societies are too high; the rise of blood pressure with age is not a natural phenomenon and should be preventable. No obvious threshold between the normal and the abnormal can be identified. Similarly, the pragmatic definition of hypertension cannot be applied in children as no randomised therapeutic trials of blood pressure reduction have been conducted. There is no level of pressure where clinical trial data dictate the use of antihypertensive drugs. Children with raised blood pressure and renal impairment are given antihypertensive drugs in the hope of preventing the development of renal failure. It would be

Table 17.2

Definitions for normal and raised blood pressure recommended by the Second Task Force on Blood Pressure Control in Children (1987).

Term	Definition
Normal BP	Systolic and diastolic BPs below 90th percentile for age and sex
High normal BP	Average systolic and/or diastolic BP between 90th and 95th percentile for age and sex
Hypertension	Average systolic and/or diastolic BP equal to or greater than 95th percentile for age and sex (measurements on at least three occasions)

unethical to withhold such treatment, even though no randomised trials are available.

In paediatric practice, a great many parameters like height and weight are considered on the basis of percentiles obtained from surveys of large numbers of individuals (see Figure 17.1). These criteria depend on the source of the individual 'normal' children but do provide sensible guidance on what levels of blood pressure require action. The USA Second Task Force on Blood Pressure Control in Children in 1987 produced a classification of hypertension and criteria for defining children as 'normal, high normal or hypertensive' (Table 17.2). These criteria are applicable to all Western countries and paediatricians should respond to them.

THE VALUE OF SCREENING

The role of well-population screening in children is uncertain. By the percentile definition of hypertension mentioned above, at all ages 5% of children will be considered to be hypertensive. No clear guidelines are available on which children should undergo routine blood pressure checks. Routine blood pressure measurement in all adults is now clearly indicated, but no information is available on the cost/benefit ratio of examining children, or on the problem of the feasibility of screening. There is no doubt, however, that some children should undergo routine blood pressure measurement in the context of either paediatric clinical practice, children's welfare clinics or the primary health care team (i.e. general practice).

Screening sick children

All children who are ill enough to be referred to a paediatrician should have their blood pressures measured at any age. In particular, children presenting with failure to thrive, those with any evidence of renal or adrenal disease and those requiring oral corticosteroid therapy need accurate blood pressure assessment. All children with diabetes mellitus should have regular blood pressure checks at least once a year.

Opportunistic screening in hospital practice

Children who are admitted to hospital for non-serious disease and, in particular, all those who are admitted for minor surgical conditions should have blood pressures measured at any age.

Screening children with high personal risk

Children who are obese have a high probability of having raised blood pressure and should have their blood pressures measured.

Table 17.3
Classification of hypertension by age group.

Age group	Significant hypertension (mmHg)	Severe hypertension (mmHg)
Newborn	Systolic BP $\geq$ 96	Systolic BP $\geq$ 106
8–30 days	Systolic BP $\geq$ 104	Systolic BP $\geq$ 110
Infant (<2 yr)	Systolic BP $\geq$ 112 Diastolic BP $\geq$ 74	Systolic BP $\geq$ 118 Diastolic BP $\geq$ 82
Children (3–5 yr)	Systolic BP $\geq$ 116 Diastolic BP $\geq$ 76	Systolic BP $\geq$ 124 Diastolic BP $\geq$ 84
Children (6–9 yr)	Systolic BP $\geq$ 122 Diastolic BP $\geq$ 78	Systolic BP $\geq$ 130 Diastolic BP $\geq$ 86
Children (10–12 yr)	Systolic BP $\geq$ 126 Diastolic BP $\geq$ 82	Systolic BP $\geq$ 134 Diastolic BP $\geq$ 90
Adolescents (13–15 yr)	Systolic BP $\geq$ 136 Diastolic BP $\geq$ 86	Systolic BP $\geq$ 144 Diastolic BP $\geq$ 92
Adolescents (16–18 yr)	Systolic BP $\geq$ 142 Diastolic BP $\geq$ 92	Systolic BP $\geq$ 150 Diastolic BP $\geq$ 98

High familial risk children

Healthy children who by virtue of family history are considered to be at high risk of having hypertension should be screened. All children of parents who have autosomal dominant polycystic kidney disease (PKD) should actively be tracked down and screened for hypertension.

These children should also undergo an ultrasound scan of their kidneys. The affected relatives of patients with PKD are frequently found to have abnormalities that require clinical action. Similarly, children of parents with phaeochromocytoma and primary hyperaldosteronism (both of which can be familial) should have their blood pressures checked.

Routine screening of all children

At the present stage of knowledge, it is not possible to justify the routine measurement of blood pressure in normal healthy children. In children under the age of 5 years, the Doppler ultrasound equipment is not generally available, so screening is hardly feasible anyway. In children aged 5–18 years, the establishment of a system for measuring blood pressure on a population-wide basis is only justifiable as a research exercise or as a study of feasibility. At the age of around 18 years, routine examination is probably worthwhile and possible, at the time of entry into higher education or prior to taking up employment.

Referral

All children with blood pressures at or above the 95th percentile need careful assessment and are best referred to a paediatrician. They may be classified as having 'significant' or 'severe' hypertension by the United States Second Task Force criteria (Table 17.3).

RECOMMENDATIONS FOR INVESTIGATING CHILDREN

Children whose blood pressures are between the 90th and 95th percentiles need investigation only if there is a suspicion of some underlying disease. Children whose blood pressures are at or above the 95th percentile always need detailed investigation and they should preferably be referred to specialised units (Figure 17.3). The method of investigation is along similar lines to those recommended in Chapters 7 and 8. Full haematological and biochemical profile, chest X-ray, renal ultrasound, ECG, urinary metanephrines or VMA and a midstream or clean-catch specimen of urine for microscopy and culture are all that is routinely needed. Further investigation depends on the results of these tests.

A good case can be made for measuring plasma renin levels routinely in all children with raised blood pressure, as this may help to detect renal hypertension.

THE AETIOLOGY OF HYPERTENSION IN CHILDREN

If the diastolic pressure exceeds 110 mmHg, it is most likely that there is an underlying renal, renovascular or adrenal cause for the hypertension. In cases where the diastolic pressure is below 100 mm Hg, it is most likely that no underlying cause will be found and, as in adults, such cases are classified as essential hypertensives.

There follows a brief classification of underlying causes that should be considered when investigating hypertension in children, with comment on each of the important clinical features.

Coarctation of the aorta

Narrowing of the arch of the aorta occurs either immediately before, at the level of, or just after, the ductus arteriosus. There may also be other cardiac defects, including patent ductus arteriosus, bicuspid aortic valves, ventricular septal defects or transposition of the great vessels. The femoral pulses may be absent or delayed and leg blood pressures are low or normal in spite of raised arm pressures. Coarctation in adults carries a poor prognosis with a high risk of myocardial infarction and subarachnoid haemorrhage. For this reason, surgical correction should be carried out as soon as is feasible and optimally at the age of about 4 years. Even with early surgery, blood pressure may not completely be normalised, so long-term follow-up is important.

Arterial disease

Hypertension may occur with congenital aortic hypoplasia. Many acquired arteritic diseases may also be complicated by hypertension. These include scleroderma, systemic lupus erythematosus, juvenile rheumatoid disease, polyarteritis nodosa and pulseless disease.

Renovascular disease

In children, renal artery stenosis is rarely congenital. Acquired stenosis is usually due to fibromuscular hyperplasia of renal or intra-renal arteries rather than atheroma. Fibromuscular hyperplasia may be seen in other vessels, including mesenteric, iliac or femoral arteries. Detailed investigation and surgical correction is mandatory. The further

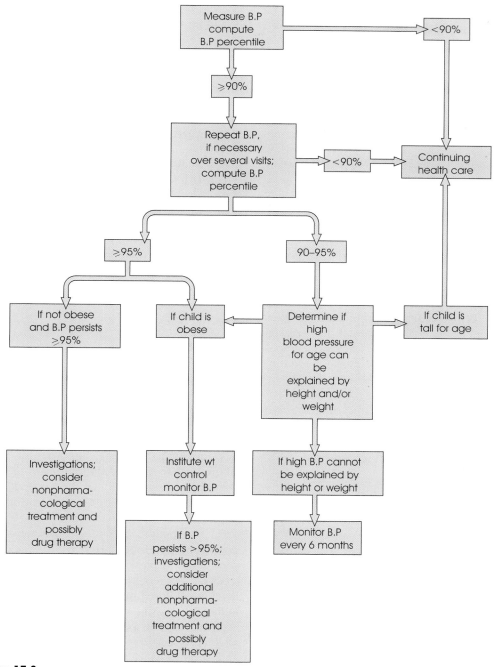

Figure 17.3
Algorithm for identifying children with high blood pressure, based on the United States Second Task Force on Blood Pressure Control in Children (1987).

investigation of renal artery stenosis is discussed in Chapter 8.

Renal disease

Renal and renovascular hypertension in children may be associated with biochemical evidence of secondary aldosteronism, with hypokalaemia and high plasma renin and aldosterone levels. These children may present with nonspecific symptoms, including general malaise and failure to grow normally or, in babies, failure to thrive. Hypertension may complicate acute nephritic syndrome, nephrotic syndrome, chronic glomerulonephritis, particularly IgA nephropathy, chronic pyelonephritis and obstructive or reflux uropathy with or without urinary tract infection. Various forms of unilateral or bilateral renal hypoplasia, including the Ask-Upmark kidney (segmental renal hypoplasia), may cause hypertension, which may be very severe. Adult-type PKD (autosomal dominant) causes familial hypertension, renal failure and subarachnoid haemorrhage. The rarer, recessively inherited, form of polycystic disease is also associated with renal failure and high blood pressure.

Very rarely, a benign renin-secreting tumour (haemangiopericytoma) may be identified. These are often small renal tumours which can usually be excised by heminephrectomy. Hypertension may also complicate renal tumours (Wilm's tumour or Grawitz tumour).

Endocrine disorders

Both primary aldosteronism and phaeochromocytoma may present in childhood. The diagnostic guidelines are similar to those described in Chapter 8. In children, hypertension may also complicate Cushing's syndrome, due to pituitary causes, adrenal hyperplasia, or corticosteroid or ACTH therapy. The very rare congenital adrenal diseases, including 11–β-hydroxylase deficiency, 17–α-hydroxylase deficiency and the apparent mineralocorticoid excess syndrome (AME) are associated with abnormal sexual development and hypertension, which is related to mineralocorticoid excess. Hypokalaemia and renin suppression, but with normal plasma aldosterone levels, are strongly suggestive of this form of mineralocorticoid hypertension. As discussed in Chapter 14, hypertension may complicate diabetes, hyperparathyroidism and possibly myxoedema.

TREATMENT

The object of antihypertensive treatment should be to reduce diastolic blood pressure to below 90 mm Hg. Careful monitoring of serum creatinine levels is necessary, since the aim of treating hypertension in children is primarily to prevent the onset of renal failure. We recommend following the algorithm in the report of the Second Task Force on Blood Pressure Control in Children (Fig. 17.3).

Salt restriction with the substitution of potassium-rich foods may be sufficient to control blood pressure in some mildly hypertensive children without renal impairment. Even in children who are receiving antihypertensive drug therapy, this dietary approach should be followed, as there is an additive effect of a low-salt diet with many antihypertensive drugs. Hypertensive children often tend to be obese, and calorie restriction should be advised where this is relevant.

Table 17.4

Paediatric doses of antihypertensive drugs. (Check manufacturer's recommendations before prescribing.)*

Class	Dose range in relation to body weight	Comments
1. **Beta-blockers**		
Atenolol	1–2 mg/kg	All beta-blockers are safe in children
Metoprolol	1–4 mg/kg	but they must not be used in asthmatics.
Propranolol	1–2 mg/kg	If there is renal failure, smaller doses should be used
2. **Thiazides and other diuretics**		
Bendrofluazide	0.1 mg/kg	These agents have long-term metabolic
Hydrochlorothiazide	2.5 mg/kg	consequences and are not usually used as monotherapy
Frusemide	0.5–2 mg/kg	For use with an ACE inhibitor
Spironolactone	1–2 mg/kg	Used only in aldosterone excess
3. **Calcium-channel blockers**		
Nifedipine	1–2 mg/kg	Safe in all hypertensive syndromes
4. **ACE inhibitors**		
Captopril	0.5–2 mg/kg	Must be used with great caution in
Enalapril	0.25–0.5 mg/kg	children with renal or renovascular disease
5. **Alpha-blockers**		
Prazosin	0.05–0.2 mg/kg	Safe in all hypertensive syndromes
6. **Centrally acting agents**		
Methyldopa	1–10 mg/kg	Safe but causes sedation
7. **Vasodilators**		
Hydralazine	1–5 mg/kg	Best avoided due to risk of lupus syndrome

*To date, there is insufficient information on the use of angiotensin-receptor antagonists (losartan) and the imidazoline receptor agonists (e.g. moxonidine) in children.

Drugs for juvenile hypertension

The same rules as for the treatment of adult hypertension apply. The thiazide diuretics, beta-blockers, ACE inhibitors and calcium-antagonists are all suitable first-line drugs (Table 17.4). The long-term metabolic consequences of thiazides make these drugs less desirable and they are also less effective in younger patients. Minoxidil causes hirsutism and is contraindicated unless all other drugs have failed. The centrally acting drugs methyldopa, clonidine and reserpine may cause undue sedation. Dosages of drugs must be corrected for the weight and age of the child as recommended in the manufacturers' literature.

The pharmacy departments of most specialised paediatric units are able to make up special elixirs containing very small amounts of the ACE inhibitors. These drugs, as well as the angiotensin-receptor antagonists, may cause over-rapid falls in pressure in children with renal or renovascular disease so they must be used with great care. On a long-term basis, however, they preserve renal function more than other drug groups in patients with diabetic and non-diabetic renal impairment.

PREVENTION

There is some evidence to suggest that essential hypertension is related to a genetically determined increased sensitivity to dietary salt. For this reason, there is a good case to be made for restricting salt intake in children with a strong family history of hypertension.

One carefully controlled study in newborn babies has shown that those given a lower salt intake had significantly lower systolic pressure at 6 months of age. A follow-up study of a number of these children, now in their teenage years, has demonstrated that those randomised to a low-salt diet at an early age still had lower blood pressures 15 years later.

Since, as mentioned above, hypertensive children, or those who have above average blood pressures, tend to be obese, weight reduction is also an important preventive approach. Children of hypertensive parents should particularly be encouraged to avoid developing obesity in the first place.

Recommendations

(a) The regular monitoring of blood pressure in all children with diabetes and those with a history of renal disease.

(b) The measurement of blood pressure and the regular follow-up of all children who have hypertensive parents.

(c) Salt restriction and, where relevant, calorie restriction in children whose parents are hypertensive.

(d) Children whose blood pressures exceed the 90th percentile should be referred to a paediatrician.

Possibilities for the future

(a) The routine measurement of blood pressure in all children of school age.

(b) Advice on salt and calorie restriction for all children whose diastolic pressures exceed 80 mmHg.

A good case could be made for restricting the salt intake of the whole population, but no studies have been carried out in children that prove this to be worthwhile. There are two studies of salt restriction applied on a population basis in adults; one showed no benefit but the other showed a reduction in the average blood pressure of the whole community.

We feel there is cause for concern that many children in the developed countries now consume large quantities of salt in convenience foods, including sausages, hamburgers and canned foods as well as snacks, potato crisps and salted nuts. The salt content of sauces and potato crisps is very high. In relation to their body weight, many children in Western countries now consume as much salt as the north Japanese, a population with the highest recorded incidence of stroke. This public health issue needs further investigation and action.

CONCLUSIONS

There is a urgent need for more information on the topic of blood pressure in children.

Most of our knowledge is based on paediatric nephrological practice and a limited number of epidemiological surveys. As the origins of essential hypertension are closely related to lifestyle factors in childhood, as well as genetic factors, more long-term research is needed on the value of preventative strategies. Children whose blood pressures exceed the 90th percentile for their age need referral to hospital specialists and detailed investigation.

FURTHER READING

Berenson GS, Wattigney WA, Bas W, et al. Epidemiology of early primary hypertension and implications for prevention: The Bogalusa Heart Study. J Hum Hypertens 1994; **8**: 303–11.

Churchill D, Perry IJ, Beevers DG. Ambulatory blood pressure in pregnancy and fetal growth. Lancet 1997; **349**: 7–10.

Dillon MJ. Investigation and management of hypertension in children. Pediatr Nephrol 1987; **1**: 59–68.

Dillon MJ. Renovascular hypertension. J Hum Hypertens 1994; **8**: 367–9.

Gruskin AB, Dabbagh S, Fleischman LE, et al. Application since 1980 of antihypertensive agents to treat pediatric disease. J Hum Hypertens 1994; **8**: 381–8.

Horn NJ. Watson AR, Coleman JE. Hypertensive adolescents detected by a school surveillance programme: a problem of obesity. J Hum Hypertens 1994; **8**: 319–21.

Report of the Second Task Force on Blood Pressure Control in Children. Pediatrics 1987; **79**: 1–25.

INDEX

Abbreviations: BP, blood pressure; CHD, coronary heart disease; LV, left ventricular; MI, myocardial infarction.